LOVE OR D...

I have been on the path to self-love for many years now but seldom have I come across a book whose voice touches me like Ani Richardson's in *Love or Diet*. Perhaps it's because Ani walks her talk and when she speaks you can feel her right beside you. Perhaps it's because she has risen from the ashes but remembers where she came from, or perhaps it's because her heart is so unconditional that you fall into it gratefully. Whatever the reason, this book is like having your BFF, your guardian angel and a box of Kleenex by your side.

We all act out our unhealthy relationship with ourselves in a myriad of ways. It doesn't matter what your poison is, what matters is that you stop hating yourself and start loving yourself, no matter what. In other words, if you must eat that box of chocolates, go ahead, but don't punish yourself for it. Ani speaks first-hand to the insidious complexities of using food to hide, numb, stuff and hurt ourselves, and with 'fierce wisdom and enduring compassion' (her words) she helps us to find the way out through self-love.

I LOVED this book and I am now and forever a fan of Ani's. For years to come, I will delight in recommending *Love or Diet* to my readers and clients. Anyone who reads it will know how fortunate they are to have Ani as their guide.
Mimi Shannon, author of *The ABCs of Self-Love – 26 Ways to Love Yourself Today* and *Self-Love The Crown Jewel*.
www.MeLoveLetters.com

I imagine that Ani's openness, sensitivity and honesty regarding her own journey will inspire, gently motivate and encourage her readers to make changes that support their own health and wellbeing. She has used her background working in nutrition and helping people with eating disorders as well as her own experience to create a supportive plan – and enjoyable read – to help readers remember how to love themselves and improve their body image and love lives.

Eve Menezes Cunningham, psychology, health and wellbeing journalist, counselor, coach, complementary therapist and owner at The Wellbeing at Work Consultancy.
www.wellbeing-at-work.co.uk

Love Or Diet is a must read for anyone who struggles with their food choices and body image. Ani Richardson's much needed holistic perspective on emotional eating sheds light on why we eat to harm rather than heal ourselves. The emotional and practical tools she shares will help you well on your way to a healthy, happy relationship with yourself and with food. Packed full of insight and inspiration, *Love Or Diet* gives you the opportunity to step off the overeating/diet roller coaster and experience self-understanding and healing on a completely new level.

Saskia Fraser, Raw Food Mentor & Life Coach. Author of *Delicious Raw Food Desserts* and *Raw Food for Winter*.
www.rawfreedom.co.uk

Dear Jessy,
Enjoy reading!
Much Love
Anix

Love or Diet

Learn to Nurture Yourself and Release
the Need to be Comforted by Food

Love or Diet

Learn to Nurture Yourself and Release
the Need to be Comforted by Food

Ani Richardson

SASSY BOOKS

Winchester, UK
Washington, USA

First published by Sassy Books, 2013
Sassy Books is an imprint of John Hunt Publishing Ltd., Laurel House, Station Approach,
Alresford, Hants, SO24 9JH, UK
office1@jhpbooks.net
www.johnhuntpublishing.com
www.sassy-books.com

For distributor details and how to order please visit the 'Ordering' section on our website.

Text copyright: Ani Richardson 2013

ISBN: 978 1 78279 091 4

A CIP catalogue record for this book is available from the British Library.

Design: Lee Nash

Cover: Monika Bienkowska
www.monides.com

Printed and bound by CPI Group (UK) Ltd, Croydon, CR0 4YY

We operate a distinctive and ethical publishing philosophy in all
areas of our business, from our global network of authors to
production and worldwide distribution.

CONTENTS

Foreword   xiv

Acknowledgements   xvi

Introduction   1

Chapter 1. Become a keeper of your inner life through
    journaling   7

Chapter 2. My journey, the path as I see it now   10
    Your own journey   18

Chapter 3. You can transform! Butterfly symbolism   22

Chapter 4. Going for gold – whys, skills and goals   30
    People eat for many different reasons
    A few words on 'why'   31
    Rambunctious resources for investigating 'why' 33
    Succulent Skills
    A word about goals   34
    What is a real woman anyway?   36
    No weight goals! Throw away your weighing scales.
        Do it now.   38

Chapter 5. The importance of self-love, nurturing and
    compassion   42
    Daily commitments for building self-love   46
    Beginning the journey, some self-love tips, quotes
    and ideas   53
    Rambunctious resources for the exploration of self-love 69

Chapter 6. You were born to sparkle and to shine   71
    Be prepared for the voice of criticism to show up when
        things get good!   76
    Real compassion can help you shine   77

Chapter 7. Being aware of thoughts   81
    Challenge your thinking   82
    Loving thoughts   85
    Accepting and loving our wholeness   86
    Rambunctious resources for the exploration of thoughts 89

Chapter 8. Take action for change   90
    Rambunctious resources for change   92

Chapter 9. Feelings and emotions   93
    It is safe to feel. All emotions are safe and acceptable. 94
    Investigate your feelings   95
    Emotions often point towards needs or desires   100
    Rambunctious resources for the exploration of feelings
        and emotions   103

Chapter 10. Investigate your food beliefs   104
    Conflict around shape change   111
    Food and sex   117
    Rambunctious resources for the exploration of sexiness 119

Chapter 11. Mindful eating   120
    Rambunctious resources for the exploration of
        mindful eating   123

Chapter 12. Assertiveness skills and learning how to have
    healthy boundaries   125
    Rambunctious resources for the exploration of
        assertiveness skills   129

Chapter 13. Learning to self-soothe without food   130
   Reduce overwhelm and stress   131
   What you can do if the urge to eat becomes strong   132
   Rambunctious resources for the exploration of
      self-soothing   133

Chapter 14. The power of gratitude, optimism and
   forgiveness   134
   Optimism   137
   Optimism could be good for the health of our heart
   Forgiveness   138
   Rambunctious resources for the exploration of
      gratitude, optimism and forgiveness   141

Chapter 15. Food wisdom   143
   Stress and food choice   144
   Nutrient density – empowered food choice doesn't
      have to be boring   145
   Blood sugar balance, mood and cravings
   Empowered eating to keep blood sugar levels
      beautifully balanced   147
   Glycaemic Index or GI   148
   Powerful Protein   149
   Fat can be fabulous   150
   Fiber   152
   Vibrant Vitamins and Miraculous Minerals
   Key points about food wisdom and a few meal and
      snack ideas   153
   Sleep impacts appetite and food choice   160
   Listen to the wisdom of your body   161
   Consider keeping a food and feelings diary   164
   Dealing with a lapse in a positive way   165
   Rambunctious resources for the exploration of
      food wisdom   166

Chapter 16. Marvelous movement and being in your
        precious body   168
    Rambunctious resources for the exploration
        of movement   169

Chapter 17. The importance of being able to ask for
    support   171

Chapter 18. Spirituality and daily connection practice   172
    The meaning of spirituality   173
    Eating as a mis-interpreted call to live more in
        the body   176
    Goddess bodies   180
    Spiritual connection as a form of intimacy   186
    Spirituality doesn't mean suddenly our lives become
        perfect with no struggle   193
    The power of 'I AM'   194
    Rambunctious resources for the exploration of
        connection   197

Congratulations!   199
    Compassion for the journey   200

References   203

Keep yourself safe

Please note: The intent of this book is only to offer general information to help you in your quest for emotional wellbeing. It is not intended as medical advice and the suggestions described should not replace the care and supervision of a trained doctor or healthcare professional. If you are taking medication or have psychological or physical problems please consult your medical doctor before you follow any suggestions in this book.

This is not a weight loss program. This book is not designed for individuals who have an eating disorder such as anorexia, bulimia or binge eating disorder or who are suffering from any other medical conditions.

If you are seeing a therapist or counselor then you might want to show them this book so that they know what you are working on and can help support you as you journey through the pages and explore your emotional eating patterns.

Much love, Ani xx

This book is dedicated to all women who struggle with emotional eating. May you be filled with loving kindness, may you be well, may you be peaceful and at ease, may you be happy. With special dedication to Chris and Freddy-dog, thank you for your unconditional love and support.

Foreword

As women, we're bombarded with images of so-called 'perfection'.

We're told to buy this: you will be better, look like this: you will be better.

We're led to believe that 'adding' things to ourselves, whether it's a pair of shoes or a pair of silicone breasts, will make us better/stronger/prettier/younger looking, when the real truth is that actually we're already pretty freakin' perfect right now, just as we are.

I often try to imagine a world where women's worth isn't measured by a size written on a dress label, where the add-ons – our clothes, the work we do, what we own, how we look, where we live – are no longer the things that validate us as women in the world – that world would rock. Hard.

But for that to happen we need to change shit up.

We need to stop looking outside ourselves for approval, for a quick fix, for the answers, and instead we need to be still, listen, and take a look inside ourselves. Girl-kind is beautiful and big hearted with our own emotion-led and intuitive inner GPS system, but currently, because society actively encourages us not to, we no longer hear our big-beat-y heart, the place where all the answers lie, and when we can't hear that, we tend to make seriously whack decisions about our lives.

When the world feels too overwhelming, I turn to food. When I feel like my heart might break when I watch the news, I eat food. When I feel rejection, pain or hurt, I turn to food. When I want to celebrate, I turn to food. When I don't stop, be still, and listen to my big, beat-y heart in a situation – good or bad – I turn to food.

Which is why I am blessed, grateful, doing star jumps o' joy that Ani Richardson has written this book.

This book matters.

As women we share stories, it's what we rock at, but it also takes deep courage to share YOUR story. But in doing so, you can encourage other women to share theirs, which is why I'm high fiving Ani for her complete honesty and truth sharing. As a trained nutritionist, g-friend knows her shit. As a woman who's struggled with emotional and binge eating, g-friend knows her shit.

In this book, Ani is a friend to hold your hand, she's someone who will help you understand what makes you emotionally eat, what you're really responding to when you choose to put certain foods in your mouth and to shine a light on any dark shadows that are stopping you from being the juicy and delicious woman you were born to be.

This book is the anti-dote to the destructive work of a gazillion pound diet industry, instead of providing a sticky plaster or yet another diet plan making false promises about how we can make ourselves better, more appealing, it will encourage you to check out of a world where being a size 0 is the Holy Grail and instead check in with yourself.

I'll be buying this book for every girl and woman I know because girl-kind needs what Ani is sharing.

Lisa x

Lisa Lister, author of *SASSY: The Go-for-it Girl's Guide to Becoming Mistress of Your Destiny*

www.sassyology.com.

Acknowledgements

There are so many people to thank, my heart could burst from the love I feel for all those who have supported me through the writing of this book. Husband Chris and gorgeous Freddy-dog, you have been there for me every step of the way, I cannot imagine my life without you both. Monika, we have known one another since I was in the womb, we are connected via our parents and grandparents; although you live far away you are always in my heart. Thank you so much for designing such a wonderful front cover for me. Lisa Lister, you believed in me and got me going with this project and then supported me throughout the journey, thank you so much. Tatiana, my darling friend, you have encouraged me through the darkest of times and shared in my brightest joy, thank you. Dad, Mum, T and Funi, I don't pretend to be the best daughter or sister, I am an ever evolving me, thanks for sticking by me as I journey through life. For all of you who have followed my work, thank you for inspiring me to continue. Rosie, I think of you often and always with love. To the woman who smiled at me as I sat weeping on the steps of my apartment bock during a really dark moment, that smile gave me the energy to stand up and begin again. You taught me that a smile can save a life, that it can create ripples that are further reaching than I could ever have imagined.

Introduction

If there was a magic spell which would allow you to eat whatever you wanted to and not put on weight, would you yearn to cast it? What would that spell, and its consequences, mean to you? Would you indulge in all the treats you had previously considered forbidden? Would you eat in public after years of secret eating, eat chocolate at every meal, have larger portions? Would you wear whatever you wanted to, hold your head up high, and skip gleefully down the street feeling light as a feather and knowing that you were sexy, attractive and wonderful, a role model to other women, envied even? Would you feel courageous and begin to magically have the life you always dreamed of, with all your worries slipping away? Would life become paradise because you were thin and eating whatever you wanted?

If you are eating to stop yourself dealing with job dissatisfaction, relationship issues, grief because of the loss of a loved one, problems with children or parents, if you are eating to prevent yourself from feeling the whole of life, the ups and downs, then being thin or losing weight will not solve those problems.

Being thin will NOT solve your problems – what feelings does that statement bring up for you? Do you want to throw this book across the room? Do you feel angry, sad, confused, cheated? Or perhaps you already know, deep down, that is the case?

Any issues that you cover up with food and eating would still be there if you were thin, nagging, pulling, needing to be looked at, accepted, worked with and healed, regardless of how thin you might be. The obsession with food covers a multitude of issues, but the beauty is that it can also be the porthole to healing. If we are willing to courageously look at what we are attempting to stuff down with food, then we can shine light on the darkness, one ray at a time. Slowly understanding our depths, discovering things about ourselves that we've kept locked up for so long is our mission here in these pages. Together we will journey toward opening, awareness, acceptance and ultimately a sense of peace with who we are.

It takes courage to step toward healing and change. Your bravery is deeply respected and acknowledged here. In this book we will gently and lovingly explore your emotional eating patterns. My own story, together with all I have learned, is woven into these pages. You are encouraged to open your heart and be fearlessly honest with yourself as you journey here, and remember that I am present, holding your hand through time and space. You are so safe and loved on this path.

When beginning this book, I had no idea that my old, dormant, emotional eating patterns would be triggered into re-appearing! Continuing to write in the face of this was a struggle. Thoughts such as 'who do I think I am to write about this topic?' started to play like a loop in my mind and that is precisely why I decided to continue writing about it, and why I am sharing this with you. The journey of healing myself went deeper through this writing process and I truly believe that I have a real compassion for your journey because of what I have been through myself over the years.

The trigger for me this time was that writing this book has been a long-term dream of mine. It doesn't surprise me that emotional eating showed up, banging at my door, as I began to write, because in the past, food was always part of a self-sabotage pattern. Any time things began to go well for me I would become terrified, start eating, numb myself and squash myself small and silent again.

It was as though I would hit a glass ceiling of how much success I would allow into my life. My unconscious belief was that I was not allowed to be successful doing something that I loved. Being happy was also not allowed by me; happiness was dangerous. This was a mirror of the beliefs of the people who were in my life in the past. My belief was that I was only allowed to be successful doing a job that I hated and that stressed me out. Being happy seemed to make the people around me jealous and nasty so that didn't feel safe either. Realizing these beliefs, being aware, making them conscious was a huge, and quite scary, step.

There are many layers to our old beliefs: cultural, familial, social, media and many more. One of the big factors for me was that, in my teens and early twenties, I didn't have many authentic friendships; my friends were prone to becoming incredibly jealous if I had any level of success or happiness. In response, instead of finding new friends, I would keep myself small in order to avoid their jealous wrath and nastiness. These were not authentic friends and, I can add, they are no longer in my life. The lessons and the love is all that I kept in my heart and took with me on my life journey. It is important for me to point out that there isn't any blame here, no finger pointing, no one to pin the responsibility to. My past friendships and relationships may well have been unhealthy but at the time I stayed in the pattern, I was as much an enabler as a victim. We do the best that we can in every moment, and in every situation, with the awareness that we have. We learn, evolve and grow along the way. During the years that my self-esteem was low it was reflected in the relationships I had in my life, they were not healthy, but as my awareness grew my friendships dissolved or changed.

There is nothing I would change in the past, even the difficult, painful parts helped to grow me to where I am now. It is true for many people that the most difficult times in life initiate the most personal growth. In the past I very much doubt that my friends were aware of our patterns or dynamics either. There is no fault here. Looking back with awareness makes it clear that what happened, happened and I am glad that I allowed change into my life. Blame keeps us small and imprisoned. Awareness, understanding, growth, evolution, compassion, courage and forgiveness set us free to love and learn. Often we cannot change outer circumstances but we can *always* change our inner response to them, we can always choose to change our thinking.

Before sorting through these beliefs, the pattern went something like this: I would have an idea for a great project, I would begin to work on it and get excited, I would share the idea with my friends, my friends would react with jealousy and would not be supportive, they would come up with horrible, snide or negative, comments or would just begin ignoring me. I would then get upset, feel abandoned and eat. Eating would numb me and I would stop working on the awesome project! Then I would also beat myself up with guilt and shame over the eating and would feel like a failure. It was one huge cycle of sabotage.

It was only after addressing the question 'who am I to shine and be successful doing something I love?' that things began to shift for me. Who am I *not* to shine? Our world *needs* shining people, people who do what they love, share their gifts in the world and encourage others to share their gifts too. Encouraging people to shine was something that I had always loved doing and now it was time to allow it for myself.

My friendships now are honest, nourishing, mutually loving and supportive; they fill me right up. The inner saboteur still shows up when I am working on projects, but I no longer head unconsciously toward food. Instead I connect with friends via the phone or email or I run to my meditation seat to allow myself to feel the feelings and get quiet. A hug with my husband and a walk with Freddy-dog also nourish me. It is no longer my belief that it is not ok to shine doing something I love. Friends help me to point my inner compass back to my own heart if things get overwhelming. We need to have people around us who are supportive and who make success feel safe.

Anyway, at the time of beginning this book, the food-saboteur showed up. However, I was conscious, and for a few days I chose to eat as a way to comfort myself. The pattern was different this time. I was eating, not binging, and there was no guilt. I was aware, I spoke to friends about it and crucially I did not give up on my project – I kept writing. It felt painful to have this saboteur show up but I believe it taught me a greater compassion for women who are experiencing these issues. After a couple of days, the pattern diminished, the saboteur left and I felt more filled with love and positivity than ever before. It is my hope and wish that this book fills you with the loving support that I intend for it to.

A key antidote to self-sabotage is self-love and self-compassion (which we'll be looking at later). Practicing self-love helps us to remember that our happiness matters and that we are so worthy of living a great, awesome life. Love yourself first and the rest will begin to take care of itself.

The words presented here are about gentle exploration into yourself and your patterns of emotional eating. You might be slim, or you might be carrying more weight than you would like. The point of this journey is to look, fearlessly, at the patterns, to uncover some of the reasons that you turn to food and how you can begin to heal this. It is not a quick-fix solution, but I assure you that you do have the power to change if you are willing.

This is a journey toward allowing more love and more joy into your life and leaving fear, and the emotional eating that goes with it, behind. Notice that I don't say 'leave it behind forever' – life is full of ups and downs. Along the way you may well turn back to emotional eating; however, it is my hope that with an open mind and heart you will feel you have a choice in the matter. You can also choose not to feel guilty or ashamed about this. Consciousness is gentle. In time you will probably find that if you do turn to food, you eat less, eat differently and stop quickly. Big, unconscious binges will probably become a thing of the past. To me, that represents true FREEDOM, you are the empowered one in the equation and food no longer takes control.

You might wonder what makes me qualified to write this book. Apart from my own personal experience, I am highly skilled in the area of nutrition and health. I am a Registered Nutritionist with specialist qualifications in eating disorders and obesity management and I also have qualifications in counseling and teaching meditations.

As all human beings are, I am complex and multi-faceted. I have come to love my complexity and my wholeness, the dark bits and the shining bright bits. To describe any woman would take an encyclopedia of space because we are all so beautifully complex, but in brief: I am a binge-reading, raw chocolate loving, meditating, motorcycle-pillion riding, tandem-cycling, dog-walking, love-loving, butterfly-adoring, wife, sister, aunt and daughter. I am a spirit adoring, poet-writing, ocean craving, sensitive and introverted woman. I am a gardening, vegetable growing, health conscious, knowing, intelligent, kosmic, nutrition hippy.

I cry, laugh, shout and giggle. I am rambunctious. I am kind, compassionate, warm-hearted and loving. I can sometimes be obnoxious and controlling about how I like the housework done. I sometimes feel anger, pain, frustration, sorrow and jealousy. I feel highs and I feel lows. I am whole. I am darkness and I am light and I am everything in between. I deeply and completely love and accept myself in my wholeness. I am perfect in my imperfections. I AM.

Chapter 1

Become a keeper of your inner life through journaling

Throughout this book you will see this symbol: ✐ which represents an invitation for you to write about your inner landscape: your feelings, emotions, physical sensations and thoughts. Often we go through life trapped in our thinking, we become walking heads, we miss the moment, we dream, we catastrophize, we let our minds run riot with scenarios and we wind ourselves up into a frenzy of mental activity.

Keeping a journal is a way to ground ourselves into the here and now. It is a way for us to record our inner experience and bring awareness to our thoughts, feelings and observations, which might have previously remained fairly unconscious. Journaling is creative expression; it is a deep way to contact our wisest Self, our deepest, innermost being. Journaling can bring personal insight and with that we can take steps toward change and growth. Writing down our thoughts can also be cathartic, a way to release past hurts or painful emotions, it can open us up and shows us a depth we didn't know existed.

A few pointers:

♥ Buy yourself a journal that really 'speaks' to you. It might be really glittery and fancy or it might be plain, elegant or grungy. The paper might be lined, unlined, have margins or borders. Go with your gut and don't listen to the critical voice which may show up saying things like 'this is stupid,' 'that's too expensive,' 'this one is way too girlie,' 'this one is too exuberant, choose something simple,' 'that's way too plain, you're supposed to choose something funky.' Just take a deep breath, look at a variety of journals and reach out for the one that feels like you!

♥ Choose a pen that is delicious to write with, or buy a pack of colored pens – you can write in any color and any size. Doodling, drawing, sticking are all allowed in journals. You do whatever you like within those pages!

♥ This is a chance for you to be fearlessly honest with yourself. The pages do not need to be shared with anyone. That choice is yours. If you are worried about someone finding the journal can you think of a safe space to store it? If you are really concerned you could keep your journal electronically in a password-protected document. Personally I feel that writing a journal by hand is more expressive and creative, there is something more powerful about writing by hand; however if that isn't an option then write freely electronically with the spell-checker off and don't worry about grammar or formatting. You need to feel safe to write without fear.

♥ If you are finding the process challenging and difficult to cope with then stop. Speak to a trusted friend or seek some help from a counselor or therapist. Keep yourself feeling safe and supported.

♥ Write every day. Take time for yourself, pause, breathe and write. It doesn't matter how long you write for, it matters just that you write regardless of the parts of you that say it is a waste of time; acknowledge those voices and write anyway.

♥ Write about anything and everything: dreams, insights, problems, joys, images, feelings, events, people, places, wildlife. Whatever comes into your heart and mind. Journaling is a great way to set up a dialogue between the mind and the heart, it gets out of our heads and into a creative, expressive state. The one thing I urge you to always do is write a gratitude list for the day – I write more

about why this is important later on.
♥ Enjoy the process! It isn't a test, you cannot do it wrong.

Chapter 2

My journey, the path as I see it now

The thing about memories is that they are subjective. We tend not to look back and see just the facts; we see a story, have feelings about the events and often give our own meanings to what we remember. The feelings and meanings come with us into the now and can impact us profoundly in the present; the memory is here with us, not stuck somewhere in the past (this is why the mystics and sages tell us there is only now, no past and no future). Looking back at the past and investigating our memories with a non-judgmental and open mind can be very healing; we might shed new light on an event and find healing in that way. Often with maturity we can look at memories with a 360 degree view, taking in the whole situation, the other people involved, how they might have felt, how their past may have impacted them and perhaps we will find compassion or a new set of eyes for seeing things with – all of this can bring sweet peace to us; we are free to re-write our story.

So, for now, this is my story as I see it. Here I include how I felt at the time and how I see things now. Looking back has helped me to understand where certain patterns came from and why I sometimes act the way I do. This understanding has meant I have been able to build support for myself in certain areas and have learned how to change my thinking and my reactions. It all takes time and I am certainly learning, growing and changing all the time!

Looking back at my childhood now I can see and appreciate that I was deeply, deeply loved. The blessed relationship I have with my mum and dad today is truly cherished, we have all grown, changed, become more conscious and are closer than ever. There is a true love between us all. For my part, I can see that this is testament to the inner work that I have done, the psychological and spiritual healing I have undertaken. I can look back now with no blame and with a healed and loving heart. There has been so much that I have learned over the years. It took me a good 10-12 years to reach this place of clarity and peace with the past and my continued conscious growth is a cherished, daily freedom, a lived and continuous journey. As the sages say, 'once you are awake you can never go back to sleep.'

When I look back, I can see that as a child I never remember feeling very close to my parents, I remember loving my mum so much and wanting her constant attention and her love but not feeling like I was really seen. My dad went away a lot on business for long stretches of time. He worked tirelessly to support our family, but as a child I didn't understand that. Mum was alone with my older brother, my younger sister and me. It must have been exceptionally tough and lonely for her. With the wisdom of age and growth, I understand my childhood in an entirely different way, but back then; I just remember desperately wanting affection and attention. I took on 'the good girl,' pleaser, mentality very early on, being mummy's little helper, always wanting to do what I could to be useful. At school I strived to be the best pupil, the helpful one, the 'teachers-pet.' Part of this early mindset involved food. I remember being praised for my clean plate, good appetite and lack of fussiness when it came to eating. I internalized not being fussy, clearing my plate and being helpful with being loveable.

My ideas about how loveable I was were very black and white, very conditional. I didn't believe that I was unconditionally loveable. If I was 'good,' helpful, quiet, polite and well mannered, then I was loveable (I might even go to heaven). If I was 'bad,' spoke back, was fussy, showed anger, then I was unlovable, unseen, nothing, a sinner (and perhaps I was destined for hell) – and in a child's mind that is very frightening.

As I grew up, it became my mission to be unconditionally

loving toward other people, I didn't yet believe I was unconditionally loveable myself but I did believe that everyone else was. The problem was, I didn't know that unconditional love does have physical and psychological safety boundaries – so during my late teenage and early adult years I allowed myself to be a doormat, I was naive and I had no balance. Looking back I see that I was desperate to be loved unconditionally, to be cherished even when I made mistakes – but the problem was I didn't unconditionally love myself, so I kept drawing unhealthy situations to me because I didn't believe I deserved better. Pointing the finger or blaming anyone, including myself, is not what I want to do here – that is a sure-fire way to self-destruction, pity and resentment. Relationship and friendship dynamics are a complex phenomenon and they evolve and change as we evolve and grow. What I have chosen to do is learn the lessons from the past and remember the love.

Anyway, I have digressed, so back to the story. Each of us begins to use food as a support system for different reasons. Early on in my life, food wasn't my 'thing.' I wasn't fussy with food and I didn't raid cupboards as a child. I ate what was on my plate with relish and gusto. As I mentioned, I do remember feeling proud that I was 'the good girl' who ate what she was given and was praised for not being fussy with food. Much later on, in my 20s, when untangling my eating issues with a therapist and in my own process, I realized that the early unconscious pattern did impact me and that I associated eating food with being praised and loved. However, until the age of about 13, I didn't really think about food, not consciously anyway. Body size/shape was something I had no concept of, we didn't watch much TV at home and my mum didn't read women's magazines, so I was spared that as a child. I spent a lot of time playing in the garden with my older brother and younger sister.

When I began secondary school, an all girls' school, I was horribly bullied. Sensitive and intelligent, I was labeled as 'nerdy.' For weeks at a time I was off school with illnesses that were medically real but which I am sure occurred due to the stress and torment I was going through (but not telling anyone because I didn't want to cause problems or trouble). Still, at this time I had no problems with food, probably because I was socially isolated. When I was around 12 years old my mum began work as a teacher, after having been a stay at home parent. She wasn't home when I got home from school and I started to help with cooking the evening meals. Again this slotted into my pattern of wanting to be helpful, to be recognized and loved. Cooking soon developed into being a creative passion for me and I found that I actually had a natural flair in the kitchen, following recipes and improvising with ingredients too.

My steady, healthy, relationship with food and eating changed when I was about 13/14. Finally I had found some friends at school and I was relieved and grateful to be free of my bullies and accepted by three lovely girls. However, being part of a friendship circle catapulted me into the world of teenaged girls and dieting. Unknowingly, the bullies had 'protected' me and kept me separate from the world of food and image issues. Suddenly I learned that 90% of my classmates were on diets, including my three new friends (one of whom was bulimic); the other 10% were the sporting heroes and had athletic bodies that were revered.

Almost overnight I decided I needed to lose weight, but I had no idea about dieting so I did nothing about it apart from listen to my friends talk. Then, a few weeks after meeting my friends, I got sick with a really nasty stomach bug that was going around the school. The chronic diarrhea and sickness, coupled with my inability to consume anything more than water and a bit of soup, meant that my weight fell. I personally didn't notice, I was too busy being unwell.

The pivotal moment came when I overheard a conversation between my mum and someone whom I loved and trusted very much. My mum had expressed concern over the amount of weight I'd lost and this trusted individual, probably in order to just stop my mum from worrying said, 'don't worry, she's getting better now and more able to eat, the weight she has lost is not the end of the world, she was starting to get a bit plump anyway.' WOW. I had never thought of myself as plump. I was only 13 and was showing signs of going into puberty; I am guessing I had begun to develop hips and a bum. I certainly don't think I was in any way 'plump.' That comment stuck in my mind, again there is no blame here but children can be incredibly susceptible to so-called throwaway comments that they overhear.

🖉 You may well have overheard many comments yourself and taken them to heart, internalized them and brought them with you as you grew into an adult.

After the sickness bug had left me, my natural feelings of hunger had returned. However, I decided to squash those hunger pangs and continue on with my water and soup, after-all it had helped me to lose weight. The hunger that I felt was intense but I somehow rode out those pains and each time I did eat a tiny amount of food, I began to feel guilt and shame, feelings I had never associated with food before. These feelings now seemed inextricably linked with food, and it would take me years of noticing and awareness before I could dismantle them and see food as food. That was it; I had begun to obsessively cut my food intake. I also began to take more notice of the diet conversations at school and I took more control over the kitchen at home – cooking elaborate meals for the family, which I didn't eat. My passion for cooking remained but I no longer allowed myself to enjoy my creations. After years of secret shame, I can now openly admit that I also made myself sick. My menstrual periods didn't begin until I was almost 16, I had no body fat to be able to produce hormones, still I had no idea how thin I was and I believed I needed to be thinner in order to be accepted and loved.

The world felt overwhelming to me at the best of times. As a sensitive introvert I just wanted to hide out by myself. From a very early age I felt quite a connection to The Mystery, the Divine, my spirituality, but it felt like I had no one to talk to about that. Having a body felt strange to me, I wanted to fly and have the feelings I had in my quiet times, the feeling of being held by something greater than me, but that was me and consumed me all at the same time. It was, and is, ineffable. Being hungry and underweight gave me feelings of being 'high' and without a body. That was a feeling I enjoyed. It felt safe, safer than being out there in the world.

At age 16, I changed schools and my food obsession quietened down, though I was still eating small portions. My obsession changed toward academic success. I did well in my A levels and went on to University, my first time living away from home. My aim was to get a first class honors degree. I wanted to prove that I was intelligent, worthy of life I guess. Working hard, I pushed myself, I got sick with a virus and then post-viral fatigue and lupus spectrum disorder (though that wasn't diagnosed until years later). However tired I was, I just couldn't seem to stop pushing myself. I did get my first class honors degree and in the process I gained an obsession with exercise and fitness as well. However, I also picked up a deep insight and passion for nutrition and health and went on to get my masters degree in nutritional medicine. Looking back, I can see that life was leading me toward where I am now.

After finishing my studies, I moved into Central London and began working as a self-employed nutrition writer, which I loved. However, I was quite isolated and hadn't really dealt with my past issues and kept going through bouts of worry about my shape and size, which was really just anxiety about deep hurts over other issues that I had squashed down. My confidence was low and I just had no love for myself. I was in pain and going through immense agoraphobia and internal distress, which I managed to hide from everyone.

A vital part of my own journey involved learning to love and care for myself, to have self-compassion and to really believe in my own right to happiness. Loving my precious self was something I always knew was important, deep down I wanted it but I wasn't sure I was allowed. Did I have permission? Wasn't it selfish to love and nurture myself? How would I even go about changing my patterns in order to love all of who I was? I was sure that people in my life would decide to leave me if I started to deeply love myself (and yes, some of them did leave).

In the past I was Ani, the girl who would do anything and everything for people she knew. 'No' was not something I knew how to say, I hadn't learned how to have boundaries and assertiveness was not in my personal dictionary. I was a give, give, giver and a do, do doer. My relationships with men were unhealthy. Many of my friendships were not authentic and I had a job where I was continually depleting myself. Being a 'good person' and a 'people pleaser' was my, somewhat unconscious, self-imposed label. The thing about self-imposed labels is that we can bust out of them when we choose to; it can cause a bit of a tidal wave amongst people who don't want you to change and grow, but it is worth it!

In 2005 I wrote in my journal that 'I find myself doing so much for other people that I am not sure I even exist any more.' My authentic self, my I AM nature was dwindling, I was lost in my overwhelming pity-party! That same year I got very, very sick (in truth, I had been unwell for a good eight years before this but never bothered to stop and do anything about it). I collapsed, I had to drag myself to the bathroom and I couldn't wash my hair because holding my arms above my head was impossibly painful and strenuous.

Carrying on my life the way I had been just wasn't an option any more. My body was holding a HUGE STOP sign up. At the time I was engaged to someone but our relationship wasn't authentic or healthy, the love wasn't unconditional, we were both in it for the wrong reasons. Well, being sick opened up my eyes – he called off our engagement, just months before the wedding. I had to leave the flat that we shared, my beautiful home. It was a wake-up call and a half. One of my closest friends also drifted away. It seemed as though now that I was unwell and couldn't be the giver and the doer and the nurturer, the un-authentic relationships around me dissolved. At the time the emotional pain was shocking; losing a friend of over 15 years felt like the loss of a part of myself, it brought up so many questions and so much self-reflection. However, after a lot of time, forgiveness (of myself as well as my friend) and openness, I gained the sweetest freedom imaginable, the freedom to be me, to grow, to change, to love myself back to life.

My self-love journey began in complete fullness. I read the books and actually did the exercises; I spent a year having therapy whilst also training to get a counseling certificate. I really took care of my body, I ate well, I exercised gently and began learning yoga and qi-gong. I nourished my soul spending time in nature, meditating daily, journaling, connecting with like-minded souls at seminars, meditation groups and healing circles. I experimented with positive affirmations, non-religious prayer and relaxation CDs. Slowly I began to make a few new, authentic friends and learned how to say 'no' lovingly and how to have boundaries. The journey wasn't always easy, but it was certainly Divine. I stayed out of a romantic relationship for 4 years whilst re-building myself. It was what I needed, and at the end of that four-year period I met Chris and we married just eight months later, on a beach, just the two of us, in Sri Lanka.

All my loving, gentle activity got me to where I am now. In reality, I want you to know there is nothing to learn. I believe that we are, already, pure love. All we need to do is allow it, fall into the arms that surround us and just let go. These parts of ourselves, like the critic and the saboteur, that created the feelings of not being good enough, or of self-loathing, are simply shadows covering the true nature of the loving light that we really are. Our task is to remove these covers in order to reveal the eternal light – the light of love that was, and always will be. This love-light is not just present in some people. It is present in all of us, and at a deeper level I believe it IS us and we are here to shine that light into the world.

It is my hope that you begin to lift the layers and reveal the light so that you can truly believe that you are love, loved and worthy of loving yourself.

Your own journey

✐ Without judgment or blame (of yourself, or anyone else) journal about your own pathway with food. Can you remember how you felt about food when you were very young and as an older child and then teenager and young adult? Do any memories or feelings stick in your mind? Can you remember any comments that impacted you? Was food used as a reward or taken away as punishment, can you remember what you made this mean? Journey as deeply as you feel comfortable. As you write, notice whether your insights about the situation become more compassionate. Can you see how everyone has their own painful 'stuff' to deal with and patterns to decipher? Can you begin to see the story from a 360-degree angle, from all sides? There is no right or wrong here, if you feel angry and hurt then that is totally valid, write about that, release those feelings from your body onto the page. When you finish writing do something nourishing for yourself – take a walk, phone a trusted friend, have a long soak in the bath, dance to your favorite music, do some yoga, meditation, painting, knitting, sewing, whatever lights you up.

So much has already been said and written about emotional, comfort eating and it is so very personal to each individual. The journey is unique to everyone and that is what I aim to capture in my writing – the uniqueness and validity of your own journey and a trust in your own wisdom. 'My own wisdom?' You might think 'I don't have any wisdom, if I did I wouldn't be reading this damned book' – that is simply not true. When we learn to get quiet and still, the voice of our deepest Self, the Wise Self, the Universal Self can be heard. This voice is knowledge and love itself and we all have access to it, in our deepest recesses we are IT. I cannot fix you or offer you a magical cure. There is nothing to fix anyway because you are a beautiful piece of perfection, you perhaps just don't see it yet. Even on a cloudy day the sun still exists, it is simply hidden from view.

Please don't see this book as a rulebook to follow, it isn't another diet book full of dos and don'ts, it is a loving guide full of supportive ideas. Keep your mind open, use your wisdom and trust that you, the wise Self that you are, can heal. Through these pages I will share my truths, some of them will ring true with you and others will not and that is fine. Trust that you will know the right actions to take for yourself at the right time. Together we can find ways to get quiet and still so that you can go deep and hear your own wisdom more clearly. As you read these words you'll also realize that you don't have to give your power away to rules, to anyone, anything or to food either. You will learn to use your wisdom-power for growth, for building self-esteem, to keep your heart secure.

Trust yourself. It is safe to listen to your own wisdom and to follow your heart. It might seem terrifying to let go of rigid thought patterns and old methods of control but that is just because you have ignored yourself for so long. Take the step toward your heart; there are no edges, only horizons. There is nowhere to fall.

The fearful voices of the critic and saboteur try to keep us safe, but we can expand and go beyond their narrow views. The voice of the wise, deep Self is never critical and never makes you feel 'bad,' guilty or ashamed. It is a loving, guiding voice that is sometimes challenging, but never cruel, hurtful or chastising. The wise voice is the you that always was, but that you learned to hide at some point in the past when you believed it wasn't safe to shine your light in the world. The world needs your light, your sparkle. Now is the time to love yourself, to choose to put yourself first, to learn to rely on your truest, wisest self for comfort and support.

Take your time. Miracles can and do happen overnight, but it is more usual for healing to happen in small, but significant, steps. Even a micro-step is a step. Each step, no matter how small, is just as much a miracle as the big leaps. The goal here is to make peace with yourself, your eating and with food, to let go of the fear and to allow love to enter all of the hurt places. Most of all it is about ending the war with your precious Self and learning how to love yourself deeply and completely and without hesitation.

The path toward healing the inner hurts and loving yourself deeply and completely isn't always easy. It is sad that we spend so much of our sacred time and energy mentally beating up on ourselves. The path towards self-love is beautiful and necessary; in fact I would say it was vital. My journey continues daily. There are still layers for me to caress and heal but it no longer feels hard to 'go there.' My heart is so open to healing, it feels natural and I relish it because each layer that is fearlessly looked at and loved is another gift to myself and to the world.

The fact that you eat for comfort, or eat to suppress your emotions, does not make you a bad person. You are simply afraid and have not yet tapped into the knowing that who you are is amazing, beautiful, whole and completely and deeply loveable. You know that deep down. You know it and you want to grasp it and live it and until you give yourself that gift and that permission to live large, then trust me when I tell you that I give you permission to SHINE.

The world needs your SHINE. Your wholeness, your authenticity. Show me your sparkly-shine! Let go of the self-judgment now. Not after you begin the healing, now. Until you can stop self-hate and self-judgment you will always head back to food. So drop it now. Yes, you may well be emotionally eating – and that really is ok – we will be gently looking at that but drop the self-hatred. Do it whilst you read this book, give yourself that gift. Read the book through, try out the suggestions; if at the end you decide that self-hatred and judgment are important in your life then you can have them back. For now I ask you to be fearless. STOP, breathe and experiment. For the duration of this book you are going to choose not to use self-hate like a cattle prod – even if, or when, you comfort eat. Instead you will be loving yourself, forgiving yourself and allowing your shine to glitter and glisten and heal you from the inside.

Chapter 3

You can transform! Butterfly symbolism

Butterflies have always represented beauty, freedom and extreme transformation for me; writing about these exquisite creatures here seems fitting and, as you will read, including a chapter on butterflies in a book about emotional eating actually makes a lot of sense. Butterflies are so captivating, the way they ride the wind gracefully and gently, landing like skilled ballerinas on the tips of flowers. It can be difficult to believe that flighty butterflies were once multi-legged, land-roaming caterpillars, which have undergone such biological and physiological metamorphosis to become winged beauties.

The American Indians view the butterfly as being a spiritual teacher of transformation and soul evolution. Butterflies are a reminder that we possess the awesome ability to change and to transform, at any given time during our lives. Old patterns and old beliefs can be dropped for new ones, we can choose to begin again, we do not have to hold onto limiting patterns or stories. This may sound simple and it is simple, but that doesn't mean that it is necessarily easy! The mind has a way of tricking us into believing that change is difficult and unnecessary even if the patterns and habits we have are harming our health, relationships and ability to live life to the full.

As well as my own personal love of butterflies, there is a deeper reason why I decided to use this potent image in my writing. When we are deeply entrenched in emotional eating patterns we often don't stop to see what our 'hunger' really represents. Sometimes, yes, we are actually, physically, hungry for food but most of the time, when we find ourselves in the cupboards mindlessly eating; we are hungry for other things, like affection, company, reassurance and love. We all have needs and often these needs go unacknowledged by us, we do not provide ourselves with what we need, let alone have the courage to ask for outside support or provision. When we forget ourselves in this way it is as though we are 'hungry caterpillars', searching outside of our own selves for answers and love, not providing ourselves with essential care and kindness. Often over-eating can be triggered by overwhelm and stress but, in fact, any emotion can be a trigger: sorrow, pain or even happiness. We'll explore some of these hungers later on. In this hungry caterpillar phase we are mainly unconscious, we do not hear the Divine Wise Self knocking at our door, we don't hear the whisper (even when it is a roar) and we don't seem able to still our racing minds for long enough to get the messages that we are being given.

In my own hungry caterpillar phase I was truly lost and in so much pain. I knew I wanted to change, to create a life of freedom and joy and I had many ideas but they felt so overwhelming that, rather than deal with them step by step, or ask for assistance, I ate to escape the feelings and got stuck in procrastination. The whole experience left me 'feeling fat,' a blanket term for 'I have feelings but I am not sure what they are.' During those times I was like one of those spiky caterpillars, I had spines for protection, I kept myself hidden away and protected, but there wasn't really any danger. I was protecting myself from living my best life! I was keeping myself small. How could I be a butterfly? I knew I needed to take the steps because the pain and fear entangled with emotional eating was blocking all the joy and love. Taking action was paramount.

To take the steps, to explore the patterns of emotional eating, we need to enter into the chrysalis, the cocoon – this is where transformation takes place from hungry caterpillar to free, beautiful butterfly.

The cocoon experience is a time of development but it is rarely a solo process. For true transformation we need to ask for help, support and guidance. In addition to this, deep thought, self-reflection and the willingness to change are key ingredients in the cocoon. It is a time to be fearlessly honest with yourself. To be able to fully investigate our emotional eating patterns we may need assistance in a variety of forms. Into my personal cocoon I took books, a psychotherapist, and lots of heart. It was a difficult process, dismantling my previous rigid structures and ways of coping and learning new ways of being. It took time and a lot of tears and lapses. In the cocoon we have to learn to let go of the past, to see things differently, to forgive ourselves, to forgive other people in our lives, to change our rigid stories, be aware of our thoughts, learn about food and allow ourselves to be truly joyful. More than anything else we have to stop hating and criticizing ourselves. We have to learn to love ourselves deeply and completely – to be gentle with ourselves, to honor our needs, to learn how to say 'no' and not feel guilty, as well as many more things, which we will explore later.

Today, I am here to provide support whilst you are in your cocoon of self-discovery. I do not have all of the answers and I cannot do the work for you but I am offering you the wisdom of my own learning, I am here to share my heart.

'The truly uncomfortable time is that in-between stage where we are becoming conscious of what doesn't work but are still caught in the middle of it. It is at this time that whatever we have been doing to numb ourselves to the pain ceases to work as well as it once did – and then we discover how much pain we are really in. As difficult as this might be, it is a necessary and powerful stage we must go through. We must have patience and compassion for ourselves, knowing that real change takes time.'
~ Shakti Gawain, *The path of transformation*

Slowly, after a lot of learning, crying, talking and exploration of my own precious Self, I began to emerge from my cocoon. This felt liberating but frightening too, as though I was leaving my security blanket. However, I knew deep down that everything I had learned was contained within me, I had forever changed. I was no longer the unconscious hungry caterpillar, I was emerging as a stronger Self, a free butterfly. Your process will be unique to you, but I assure you that you too will fly.

Emergence from the cocoon is not to be rushed; we can take our time, gently pushing through into the outside world with help and support. To emerge as a butterfly deserves celebration. It is a time to share the joy of our explored and liberated selves with the world around us! As a butterfly we are conscious of our emotions, thoughts and feelings. We have learned to breathe and to pause before we react. We have a toolkit in place so that if we are triggered or overwhelmed we don't simply self-destruct. We can learn to fly, to shine, to be the best of who we are. Remember, we can also land in the safety of a gorgeous flower and drink the nectar, here we learn more, get more support, take time out, breathe and transform further. As a butterfly it is not that we are cured, but we are healed. We have peace, we have tools. Our inner self has been un-recognizably changed from the hungry caterpillar. As a butterfly we might still emotionally overeat at times, but the eating has less power, we don't feel guilty, we recover more quickly, we have ways to help ourselves and, because we have cultivated deep self-love, we know that there is nothing to fear. We are love; we are Letting Outrageous Vitality Emerge!

As a butterfly, I began to do work that I loved; I gained new qualifications, made new friends and began dressing the way I wanted to dress. I allowed myself to feel happiness and joy as well as not suppressing sorrow. Instead of living in a black and white world I began to live the rainbow.

My support is loving, kind, compassionate and safe. As I said before, I cannot take the journey for you – it wouldn't work, but as the story below illustrates, the journey is so worthwhile and I am here encouraging you to take your steps.

A man found a cocoon of a butterfly. One day a small opening appeared. He sat and watched the butterfly for several hours as it struggled to squeeze its body through the tiny hole. Then it stopped, as if it couldn't go further. So the man decided to help the butterfly. He took a pair of scissors and snipped off the remaining bits of cocoon. The butterfly emerged easily but it had a swollen body and shriveled wings. The man continued to watch it, expecting that any minute the wings would enlarge and expand enough to support the body, neither happened! In fact the butterfly spent the rest of its life crawling around. It was never able to fly. What the man in his kindness and haste did not understand: The restricting cocoon and the struggle required by the butterfly to get through the opening was a way of forcing the fluid from the body into the wings so that it would be ready for flight once that was achieved. Sometimes struggles are exactly what we need in our lives. Going through life with no obstacles would cripple us. We will not be as strong as we could have been and we would never fly.

Transformation can feel incredibly uncomfortable, as well as necessary and right. Do not enter into the illusion that something which feels imperative and 'right' will just flow naturally. Of course it can, but in most cases old habits form walls to our forward movement. Our challenge, as uncomfortable as it may be, is to rise above that wall, to begin to slowly challenge those old habits one by one, with compassion and love. In her book, *Entering the Castle*, Caroline Myss writes:

You may struggle all the way into the cocoon, but you cannot sidestep a cocoon experience if it is time for one in your life. You can choose, however, how to experience the cocoon. You may be able to draw comfort from recognizing that you are preparing for emergence into the light, rather than fear that you are alone in a dark, lonely place. To be able to illuminate your most painful moments – or days or months – with the mystical truth that you are living a transformation in progress brings God into the walls of your soul.

Knowing that the journey of transformation is challenging for everyone can help you to recognize that you are not alone, everyone faces hurdles and blocks, you are not flawed in the slightest. Know that on this journey you may slip and that is ok. Everyone uses food emotionally at some times. Everyone. You are not 'bad' if you trip. It is time to leave self-hate at the door and crawl into the cocoon.

I invite you now to take the journey. Are you ready to step into the cocoon?

In order to get the best from this book you first need to make the solid decision that you are ready and willing to change. You need to understand that it does take motivation and effort and although this information is here to support you, as I am, the real change is down to you. It is not always easy but it really is worthwhile. Take a look at some of the questions below, these are there to help you tune into how ready you are and what kinds of blocks or resistance might come up for you. The book will still be useful to you even if you cannot dedicate your whole self to this journey, as reading it will plant the seeds that can be watered and grown, but to get the most out of the words here you need full readiness, willingness, compassion and love for yourself.

🖉 Take your journal to a quiet space, go through the questions below and be honest with yourself. There is no score to calculate, these questions are simply there to help you to feel into yourself, to highlight any blocks and resistances that you might need to crack open with a loving and compassionate heart.

♥ How motivated are you to explore, and free yourself from, your emotional eating patterns?

♥ How certain are you that you will stay committed to your decision to read this book and take your own steps toward change?

♥ How supportive are the people around you? Will they be pleased with your decision to want change? (People often find change frightening.)

♥ How supportive is your life circumstance at the moment – will you have the time to dedicate? Are you very stressed at work or in your relationships?

♥ Do you have a comfortable, quiet and safe place that you can dedicate to your journey? A quiet room where you won't be disturbed, where you can retreat to be still?

♥ How is your health? If you are suffering with a long term physical or mental/psychological condition then it is best to check with your medical doctor before embarking on any kind of lifestyle change. If you are seeing a counselor or therapist perhaps you can take this book to show them what you are going to be working on.

♥ How is your mood? If you are feeling very low, depressed or anxious then this could interfere with your ability to make changes.

♥ Are you ready to change? For me it was difficult to be ready to be joyful in front of my family and some of my friends – these relationships seemed to thrive on misery and any joy was frowned upon or invoked jealousy. I had to make the decision to change anyway and allow myself to shine my light. Yes, I lost some friends but my family seemed to magically change with me!

♥ Do you sleep well? Adequate sleep is really important to help you on this journey. Can you commit to going to bed earlier if you need to, or changing your sleep habits?

♥ Is there anything else you need to consider, anything that might make this journey difficult?

♥ Can you find room in your life for yourself?

Are you ready to GO FOR IT? If you want to deeply explore yourself and your emotional eating patterns then please continue. I am so, so proud of you and your decision to take this journey. I send you my deepest love and I want you to know that I am here, beyond the bounds of time and space, supporting you.

Chapter 4

Going for gold – whys, skills and goals

People eat for many different reasons

As someone who eats emotionally, you may eat for all of the reasons below and many more. Now is NOT the time to feel guilty about this and there is no need for shame or judgment. Negative thinking around this issue is fear's way of holding you back from change. Be gentle with yourself as you explore your eating patterns. Be fearlessly honest with yourself.

🖉 We all eat for different reasons; here are just a few examples. See if you can think of some more:

- To satisfy true physical hunger;
- For fun;
- To manage feelings such as sadness, boredom, overwhelm and frustration;
- To block feelings;
- To create feelings – such as excitement;
- To celebrate events such as birthdays;
- As a way to interact with others and fit in;
- Out of habit at certain times of the day;
- As a reward;
- To self-soothe;
- Out of loneliness.

Some individuals may turn to alcohol, prescription drugs or illegal drugs in order to cope with their emotions. On many occasions, and in many conversations, I have heard it said that people who struggle with various food issues, and those who use food to deal with stress and emotions are in a difficult position because they cannot 'give up food' in the way that an alcoholic can stop drinking, for instance. This mindset is simply not an empowering one. It is true that an alcoholic can give up drinking, but if they don't deal with the underlying issues then they will be forever teetering on the edge of relapse. You have the opportunity to really uncover and break open your emotional eating patterns and learn to cope in an environment where food is plentiful and needed for life, and that is truly empowering! Yes, food is every-where but it is also your porthole into healing. It is not an enemy. As you explore yourself you may well find that your relationship to food changes, particularly your relationship to specific foods. Your cravings may reduce or disappear, your tastes may change, and all kinds of miracles are ready to be released.

A few words on 'why'

There has been a lot of study in the psychology field as to why people emotionally eat. All reasons are valid. Some of the reasons that have been investigated include:

- Genetic factors;
- Availability of food;
- Poor food choices that can lead to cravings;
- Lack of activity;
- Psychological barriers. It is important to know that change is difficult for the majority of people. Emotional eating served a purpose once (for example when you were a child and lacked other coping mechanisms) and now it might have become a habit or a pattern that is no longer needed but change seems frightening and daunting. Sometimes people eat to satisfy other people, this stands in the way of change, as there can be fear about upsetting or losing the person in question;
- Due to trauma (such as abuse or neglect) in childhood or adulthood, food becomes a way of self-soothing;

- Lack of knowledge about other coping mechanisms to deal with stress or emotion;
- Biological/physiological factors. Certain foods can impact the chemistry of the body and brain leading to short term pleasant sensations. If you don't have any other coping mechanisms to deal with e.g. upset, stress or overwhelm then food becomes a means to make you feel better (at least in the short term until the effects wear off and you feel miserable).

In this book we are not going to overly concentrate on the whys. The aim here is to look at positive ways to change behavior away from using food for emotional comfort. We will be investigating a variety of skills that can help you to cope better so that you turn to food less often for comfort.

If you have read the above list and feel that you need to discuss the reasons why you turn to food for emotional support then I would recommend you find a fully qualified counselor/therapist to work with. This might feel frightening but please rest assured that it is a safe and loving decision for you to make. You can call a number of therapists to see how you feel about them before committing to working with them. Remember you will be paying them, so interview them! Some therapists are specifically qualified to work in the area of addiction and eating disorders; please visit the British Association for Counseling and Psychotherapy – here you can search for qualified therapists in your area:

http://www.bacp.co.uk/seeking_therapist/right_therapist.php

My own personal experience with therapy has been fantastically healing. The therapist I saw was a psychosynthesis therapist, whom I chose specifically because of her use of the transpersonal, or spiritual, in her work, and also due to the use of visualizations and creative expression. There are many types of therapy available, so do some investigation before making your choice. Listen to your heart's needs.

Rambunctious resources for investigating 'why'

♥ *Understanding Your Eating, How to eat and not worry about it.* By Julia Buckroyd.
♥ *French Toast for Breakfast. Declaring peace with emotional eating.* By Mary Anne Cohen.
♥ *You can't quit 'til you know what's eating you. Overcome overeating.* By Donna LeBlanc.
♥ *It's not about food. Change your mind, change your life, end your obsession with food and weight.* By Carol Emery Normandi and Laurelee Roark.

Succulent Skills

Here are some skills that we are going to investigate and learn about in this book:

♥ The importance of self-love, self-nurturing and self-compassion for building healthy self-esteem.
♥ How to investigate our own thinking in order to prevent self-defeating thoughts that can lead to emotional eating.
♥ Flexibility skills to help you get comfortable with change so that you can learn to get out of the habit of turning to food.
♥ How to handle feelings and emotions.
♥ How to eat mindfully.
♥ Assertiveness skills and how to handle challenging people.
♥ How to self soothe without using food.
♥ Food wisdom. Learning about how certain foods really can impact the mood and cravings.

- ♥ How to deal with a lapse in a positive way.
- ♥ Why movement is a great friend! (Please note that I don't use the word exercise, it sounds so boring and like a chore!)
- ♥ The importance of being able to ask for support.
- ♥ Having a connection practice – to connect with your deepest Self, this can be called Spiritual Practice.

A word about goals

Be reasonable with your goals. This is a journey of self-exploration. As mentioned earlier it is not about weight or weight loss, although weight loss may be a by-product. This journey is about self-discovery, the willingness to change and to take action. Setting a goal like 'I am never going to emotionally eat again' is not helpful because ALL people use food as an emotional support at some point.

All or nothing thinking is destructive. Life is not black and white – thank goodness because there are so many colors in the rainbow to experience! The first goal is to be willing to explore your emotional eating patterns with a wide open, gentle, heart and to be willing to take action toward change. Your journal will help you track your progress as you take steps on the path toward peace with emotional eating.

It is important to remember that being thin doesn't equate to wellness. Wellness is a state of being in healthy balance of mind, body, emotions and spirit which results in a feeling of 'being well.' Factors that contribute to being healthy and happy are individual and varied but may involve concepts such as: nutrition, exercise and other health practices; spirituality; psychology or counseling to explore the mind; work; money and security; creativity; leisure; family and social support.

Wellness for me is a progression toward being my best possible self, doing my best not to compare myself to others and regularly checking in with my own feelings to see if I am making choices that empower me, those around me, and the environment. Living life to our fullest potential is not something that we often do, fear is a tyrannical ruler! Now is the time to break free and break through, living our best lives is allowed, it is needed and it is a beautiful gift to ourselves and the world.

🖋 What does wellness mean to you?

In order to find our personal wellness we need to look within and not be swayed by the media, which is, frankly, just a circus. Women are shamed for being too thin or too fat, they are praised for losing weight, unless they lose 'too much' weight and then they are vindicated, or they are ridiculed for putting it on. There is much talk about 'real' women being curvy, but this is just another media trick. We are all REAL women; we come in all shapes and all sizes. Comparison breeds eating disorders, we think we have to be this or that, but the true challenge in life is to be who we are, and this can change constantly, it is fluid and flowing, not some rigid idea. For a truly powerful look at body shape and acceptance I would highly recommend reading Chapter 7 of *Women Who Run With The Wolves, myths and stories of the wild woman archetype* by Clarissa Pinkola Estes. The chapter is entitled 'Joyous Body: The Wild Flesh' and includes a story about La Mariposa, Butterfly Woman.

'There is no 'supposed to be' in bodies. The question is not size of shape or years of age, or even having two of every-thing, for some do not. But the wild issue is, does this body feel, does it have right connection to pleasure, to heart, to soul, to the wild? Does it have happiness, joy? Can it in its own way move, dance, jiggle, sway, thrust? Nothing else matters...Wild Woman shows up in many sizes, shapes, colors, and conditions. Stay awake so you can recognize the wild soul in all its many guises.'
~ Clarissa Pinkola Estes

What is a real woman anyway?

We all come in different shapes and sizes. It is about time we celebrated that, celebrated one another and stopped wasting precious time and energy on envy or comparison. I am 5'7" and I am naturally quite slender (not skinny). At the height of my stuffing episodes I was bigger but it wasn't the weight or shape that upset me (although in my mind I was huge), it was the fact that I was binging when I wasn't hungry, I was giving my power away to an outside force, food, in the belief that it would 'save me' from myself. When really, what was needed was for me to love myself, to look within, to use the empowered self that is, and always was and will be, precious and there for me. So, I am not a large girl, I don't weigh myself and don't own a set of scales so I have no idea what my weight is. I have long-ish legs, small breasts and a bigger bum and hips in comparison to my top-half, I am not really curvaceous. I am beautiful in my own way.

When you read that I am slender what do you feel? Do you think 'she won't understand,' 'she's lucky,' 'she's a bitch?' Well, as mentioned earlier I have been through eating disorders (anorexia and bulimia), depression, and emotional eating episodes, I have a deep compassion for your struggle. I also have a progressive autoimmune condition, which could attack any organ of my body and impacts me on a daily basis. Do you still think I am lucky to be slender? Can you see it isn't all about size? We are all human, all perfect in our imperfections. We all feel pain and we all know joy. We all have our own struggles to go through; no one is more of less worthy of love than we are. Let's set aside the comparisons and begin to celebrate and support one another rather than simply looking at outward appearance.

Comparison is painful; it breeds self-hatred and reduces compassion, for ourselves and others. Comparison also makes us less available, to ourselves and to the people in our lives – because it takes up so much time and mental space to constantly compare! It is an illusion to think that 'when I am thin I'll be happy' that is simply not true. We can all choose happiness and life in the now. I have been through really depressive episodes, just like you, pain and strife, just like you. None of this has anything to do with size or shape.

When we begin to love ourselves, when our emotional eating calms down, our bodies find their balance. Each of us will have a different, unique, shape and size and that will also change over time. When you love yourself deeply and completely, when you embrace the whole of who you are, then you will find a sweetness that has nothing to do with size.

Stop comparisons now. Stop reading those magazines that tell you there is something wrong with the way you look. Skinny people, thin people, curvy people and large people may or may not be binge eaters or have issues with food. The challenge for each of us is to get back to ourselves, love ourselves, love our unique bodies and find a peacefulness within. When self-love is our focus we naturally choose nourishing foods and beverages and our bodies naturally love us right back.

Go on, I dare you. Love yourself. The only thing stopping you is you.

During my writing process I was reminded of the Shakespeare play, *The Merchant of Venice*. In the play Shylock makes a speech about being ridiculed and hurt simply because he is a Jew. He says,

Hath not a Jew eyes? Hath not a Jew hands, organs, dimensions, senses, affections, passions? Fed with the same food, hurt with the same weapons, subject to the same diseases, healed by the same means, warmed and cooled by the same winter and summer, as a Christian is? If you prick us, do we not bleed? If you tickle us, do we not laugh? If you poison us, do we not die?

We are all women. We all laugh. We all cry. We all feel pain. We all know joy. Is it not time now to stop compartmentalizing ourselves by our shape and weight? It really is time for us to celebrate one another and stop the fanfare of envious comparisons, ridicule and hurt.

✎ What does the term 'real woman' mean to you? Are your thoughts on this matter empowering or dis-empowering? Could you begin to change your thinking and expand your notions about what being a woman really means to you?

The issues with food are deep. It's as though; if we do not fit the ideal then we must be fundamentally flawed. Who set the 'ideal?' You can reset your own ideals. It is not true that you are somehow 'bad,' 'wrong' or whatever if you are not a waif. It is simply not true that men all want the same thing in a woman, and if they did then so what? YOU have to love on yourself. Marry yourself internally. When you start eating due to true physical hunger signals and listening to what the body wants you will change shape and eventually your body will settle into a place of peace, and that place is different for every single person. Short, tall, slim, curvy, you will find a place where your body sighs and all is well and you won't care that you are not a size six with huge breasts or whatever the particular penchant is that day. Women are women, we are beautiful and we are different and we have to rock the body we have.

No weight goals! Throw away your weighing scales. Do it now.

Oh for the Love of your Divine Inner Goddess, please, please, throw away those damned bathroom scales! I am totally on my knees begging you to take this action.

✎ What do you think those scales are going to tell you? That you are now worthy enough to wear what you want to wear? Do what you want to do? Say what you want to say? Walk and talk how you want? Are they going to give you permission to love yourself?

Your weight can vary up to 6lb depending on where you are in your menstrual cycle. You may also notice that you weigh more at the time of the full moon – because of water retention, and no, I am not making that up. The moon is responsible for controlling the tides of the sea; do you not think it might also be impacting the water balance in your own body? Water weighs. The moon and menstrual cycles also seem to impact appetite for many women too. Keeping a journal and tracking moon phases can be an interesting and informative exercise.

Give yourself, your precious, precious self, a break. Instead of weight you can use other markers to track your health. Some people like to use blood pressure as a measure, as they become healthier it drops into the healthy range. Other people like to use fitness as a measure – go to your local park, see how long it takes you to walk around it once. Then each week, or two weeks, you can time yourself again and see if you're walking quicker. Or choose another goal e.g. each week when you go to the super-market try a new fruit or vegetable, or make it your goal to reach 5+ portions of vegetables and fruit a day.

Set self-love goals, we'll be delving into self-love in the next section. Stick post-it notes up which say 'I love you' or 'you are beautiful' or 'I am so precious.' Do something every single day to love on yourself. Make that non-negotiable. Read books that fill you with wonder and awe and nourish your soul. Write your own stories, journal, share your feelings with other women. You are so worthy of self-love now, not when the number on a scale tells you so.

🖋 Journal about some personal goals, non weight loss goals!

We run to the scales for re-assurance, or validation – they are inanimate objects, they cannot tell you your worth. You are so precious and fabulous; don't look to the scales for love, because they are just not able to give it to you. YOU, you can give yourself so much love, just be willing. Make the choice to treat yourself like the amazing woman that you are. Do it now, do it every day. Don't wait for the perfect weight because that's just an illusion too. More often than not, women say that the more they weigh themselves the more they emotionally eat. It is just a habit and habits can be broken and new, more loving, ones can be formed.

Do it, chuck the scales out. Or give them to a charity shop, destroy them or think of something else to ritually release them from your home. Not owning a set of scales is liberating, it will give you space to breathe.

Put a self-love plan into action using the information in the next section. I'm cheering you on, pom-poms and all. Don't rely on the scales to tell you what and how you are going to eat that day, or how much, or what time, this kind of control ultimately leads to out-of-control binges and eating because you begin to deprive yourself, or you don't listen to the wisdom of your highly-intelligent body. Get silent, get still and listen to that voice of wisdom, which is your own truest Self.

🖋 Weigh your life with the scales of passion. How passionate are you today? What can you do to feel life flowing through you today? Is there a hobby you want to try? Do you need to play?

Letting go feels scary and it may take a bit of time to get used to actually relying on your body, but it will tell you when it wants food and you can trust that, it doesn't have to be at a specific time, it will be when it is right for you. Would you tell a child that they were not worthy of love that day if the scale said x, y, or z? Of course not. You are a precious child of the universe. You deserve your love and affection now.

Give yourself to this process. During the time it takes for you to read this book take space to practice self-love and put into action the other ideas in this book. This is the bedrock for building a healthy you. You have probably been 'battling' with food, weight, and shape issues for years – so commit to this new, loving practice. No battle. No bashing yourself with your words or weighing yourself or making this process about weight at all. After reading this book if you don't feel more peaceful within, and ready to make loving yourself a lifetime priority then you can go back to your old methods. Give yourself this time; it could make the rest of your lifetime feel amazing.

Chapter 5

The importance of self-love, nurturing and compassion

Originally this book was due to start in an entirely different place, but as the writing process evolved, it became apparent that beginning with a healthy self-love was vital. It seems to be the bedrock, the foundation that is necessary for healing on so many levels.

If you truly loved yourself you would treat yourself like the beautiful, precious human being that you are. You would treat yourself like your own best friend. You would stop beating yourself up for using food to deal with your emotions. In fact, I suggest that this beating business actually causes us to continue with the emotional eating because we end up feeling so 'bad' and horrible that we are drawn again to the comfort of food. Remember that all of the negative self-talk is not who you are, it is the voice of the inner critic and the saboteur (we'll be looking at the critic and saboteur later when discussing thoughts and thinking). Who you are is perfect love.

We may have built up a persona of being the 'nice' one, the pleaser, the kind and gentle being who is self-less with no needs, always there ready to assist. The truth is – this is a lie. We are not always nice or kind, we are violent and nasty with ourselves, we hurt ourselves with food, we squash down our own needs and veil them with binges. We do this because on some level we do not believe we are worthy of loving our own precious selves or giving ourselves the attention that we give to others. Somewhere, deep down we are angry at how we give ourselves away and leave no time for us, but we don't acknowledge our needs or our anger because we have been taught this is wrong. Food becomes the cover. Then we have more ammunition against our preciousness because we feel the weight of guilt over being an emotional eater, it is as if we have proven ourselves right. We decide that we are bad, bad people.

If we can recognize this faulty belief we are on the road to recovery and healing. We can make the choice to change. We can decide to begin the journey toward self-love. When you truly learn to love yourself you can be gentle and kind to yourself and your needs. If you slip up with your eating you'll give yourself a compassionate hug and find peace again rather than beat yourself up and then eat more and more in an unconscious vicious cycle.

Most of us have not been taught the highly important skill of self-love and so we have to start this learning from scratch, which can seem awkward at first, or just downright ridiculous. However, it is vital that you give yourself this gift of learning because life really is sweeter when you realize you can go within to get your needs met and you can love yourself deeply and completely as a perfectly imperfect, wondrous human being. It will open you up to loving more deeply in the world too. If you are skeptical then just experiment, see what happens when you speak to yourself as though you were a precious being (because you are one!). Then speak to yourself with your usual critical, harsh voice; which feels better in your heart?

'Offering ourselves such care might feel strange and unfamiliar at first. Sometimes extending compassion to ourselves in this way feels downright embarrassing. It can trigger a sense of shame about being needy and undeserving, shame about being self-indulgent. But this revolutionary act of treating ourselves tenderly can begin to undo the aversive messages of a lifetime.'
~ Tara Brach. *Radical Acceptance*

Loving my precious self was something I knew was important,

deep down I wanted it but I wasn't sure I was allowed. Did I have permission? Wasn't it selfish to love and nurture myself? How would I even go about changing my patterns in order to love all of who I was? I was sure that people in my life would decide to leave me if I started to deeply love myself (and yes, some of them did leave). I was Ani, the girl who would do anything and everything for people she knew. 'No' was not something I knew how to say, I hadn't learned how to have boundaries. Give, give, giving and do, do doing was my modus operandi. I had unhealthy and unloving relationships with men. Many of my friendships were not authentic and I had a job where I was continually depleting myself. Being a 'good person' a 'people pleaser' was my self-imposed label.

It became obvious that carrying on my life the way I had been just wasn't an option any more. So I began the self-love journey in complete fullness. As I mentioned earlier I read the books and actually did the exercises, I spent a year having therapy whilst also training to get a counseling certificate. Taking really good care of my body became important, I ate well, I exercised gently and began learning yoga and qi-gong. My soul was nourished by spending time in nature, meditating daily, journaling, connecting with likeminded souls at seminars, meditation groups and healing circles. I experimented with positive affirmations, non-religious prayer and relaxation CDs. Slowly I began to make a few new, authentic friends and learned how to say 'no' lovingly and how to have boundaries without feeling tremendous guilt for counting my needs as important.

In reality, I want you to know that I truly believe there is nothing to learn. We are, already, pure love. These parts of ourselves, like the critic and the saboteur, that created the feelings of not being good enough, or of self-loathing, are simply shadows covering the True Nature of the loving light that we really are. Our task is to remove these covers in order to reveal the eternal light – the light of love that was, and always will be.

This love-light is not just present in some people. It is present in all of us, and at a deeper level I believe it IS us and we are here to shine that light into the world. As you begin to love and care for yourself, you begin to lift the layers and reveal the light so that you can truly believe that you are love, loved and worthy of loving yourself.

When you learn self-love you realize that you have great wisdom within yourself. Over time you will probably find that you eat to cover your emotions less and less and the times that you do emotionally eat you will be conscious, you will choose to eat as a response to a felt emotion, you will enjoy the food more, be more present to the tastes and textures and won't continue on to extreme emotional eating that lasts days on end. Be really compassionate with yourself on this self-love journey. Having support from a friend, therapist, counselor and even online communities can be very helpful.

Create a daily practice of radical self-love. Make this non-negotiable. Included below is an idea that you could use but feel free to form something scrumptious for yourself. Do it so that your heart feels loved. Begin now. It may seem really strange, strained and false at first but stick with it, over time it will become natural. You are precious, as precious as any other being, you are worthy of this.

It would be easy to just read this chapter and think yeah, I could do that, I'll start at another time, but another time is too late. Now is that time. Commit to self-love whilst you read this book and then see how you feel after that. See if you notice changes within you and outside of yourself. Keep journaling, keep yourself open to awareness – there are gems to be discovered on your journey.

Make posters that say 'I love you,' put them up. Put them on the kitchen cupboards and the refrigerators and the front door – this may help you tune into consciousness and help break the habit of unconscious eating. It may help you to get a dialogue going between your head and your heart. Don't just think about doing it, do it!

✎ In your journal, write some answers to the following questions: if you really loved yourself how would you live? How would you dress? Walk? Talk? Eat? Play? Make love? Can you see that is only a micro-second away? All it takes is a choice, a choice to begin self-love. You can be that person now. The other way is violence toward yourself with words and thoughts. It is self-criticism and negativity and a constant returning to emotional eating.

Here are some ideas for daily commitments to help you build a foundation self-love, do these until it becomes natural and comfortable to love on yourself each and every day. Or build your own daily self-love program and commit to it for at least 21 days.

Daily commitments for building self-love

♥ Before you jump out of bed and start your day say, out loud or inwardly, 'Today I am willing to learn to love myself deeply and completely.' Take a minute to breathe and feel your body. Imagine your heart filling up with pink light and then imagine that soft light of love travelling into every cell in your body and transforming your thoughts into loving ones. Following this practice say, 'I deeply and completely love and accept myself and I commit to practicing radical self-love today.' Notice any thoughts or feelings that come up. If these are negative you can say to yourself, 'even though I feel angry/frustrated/sad/self-critical/stupid/phony I choose to deeply and completely love and accept myself anyway.'
♥ Do something for yourself each day that is completely loving and nurturing. This can be something small or large e.g.

- take time to rub lotion into your hands or body,
- take a bubble bath,
- allow yourself to really enjoy your shower,
- take a walk in nature,
- eat a piece of fruit or drink a delicious smoothie and really taste it,
- say 'no thank you' to something you really don't feel you want to do,
- say 'yes please' to something you really do want to do but wouldn't normally allow yourself.

If you get really stuck then close your eyes, breathe love deeply into your heart and ask, 'what would love do?' See if an answer comes.

♥ Throughout the day repeat to yourself, 'I deeply and completely love and accept myself.' [I have an app on my phone where I can program in positive affirmations, they buzz onto my screen every couple of hours and remind me to pause and breathe in some love for myself.]

♥ Each day name one thought, belief or behavior you need to give up that day to allow self-love to shine, e.g.
- 'I'm not worthy,' 'I always mess up,' 'My life is awful,' 'I'm too short, thin, fat, tall, pale etc.'
- Over-working, over-giving, people pleasing.

During the day if you catch yourself inside a negative belief, or unhealthy behavior pattern, STOP, BREATHE deeply and then say, 'Even though I feel _____ I deeply and completely love and accept myself.' Choose to love yourself anyway, bring your attention to your breath and relax as best you can.

♥ Each day spend at least 15minutes in silence with no TV, radio or music. You will need a journal that you can write in, or just a stack of paper. Start by writing anything that comes up for you; don't judge it just write – thoughts, feelings, conversations you've had that impacted you.

Then write what you are proud of for today, what did you do that you feel really good about? When you are ready to finish write at least five things that you are grateful for. Really focus on gratitude, are you grateful for your warm bed? Hot running water? Your best friend, lover, mother? Are you grateful that you allowed love into your heart?

♥ Before you go to bed read the acceptance quote, below, and say, 'I deeply and completely love and accept myself.' If you are really struggling with the sentence, 'I deeply and completely love and accept myself,' and simply cannot believe it yet, then start with 'I am willing to learn to deeply and completely love and accept myself.'

Acceptance Quote:

I accept myself completely.
I accept my strengths and my weaknesses,
my gifts and my shortcomings,
my good points and my faults.

I accept myself completely as a human being.
I accept that I am here to learn and grow,
and I accept that I am learning and growing.
I accept the personality I've developed, and
I accept my power to heal and change.

I accept myself without condition or reservation.
I accept that the core of my being is goodness
and that my essence is love,
and I accept that I sometimes forget that.

I accept myself completely, and in this acceptance
I find an ever-deepening inner strength.
From this place of strength, I accept my life fully and

I open to the lessons it offers me today.
I accept that within my mind are both fear and love,
and I accept my power to choose which I will experience as
    real.
I recognize that I experience only the results of my own
    choices.

I accept the times that I choose fear
as part of my learning and healing process, and
I accept that I have the potential and power
in any moment to choose love instead.

I accept mistakes as a part of growth,
so I am always willing to forgive myself and
give myself another chance.

I accept that my life is the expression of my thought,
and I commit myself to aligning my thoughts
more and more each day with the Thought of Love.
I accept that I am an expression of this Love.
Love's hands and voice and heart on earth.

I accept my own life as a blessing and a gift.
My heart is open to receive, and I am deeply grateful.
May I always share the gifts that I receive
fully, freely, and with joy.

~ Author unknown

Writing this book became a spiritual odyssey for me. It is evident
that emotional eating is about food – but it is not just about food.
It is about the body – but it is not just about the body. It is clear
that the path to healing is about finding a deep, unshakeable love
for ourselves. We have to make the fearless choice to follow the

call of our True Nature to shine, to allow ourselves to be all that we can be. It is my belief that Spirit, our True Nature (God, Goddess, Tao, whatever you wish to call it) is always calling us. We already are 'all that' but part of us doesn't believe it and we choose to stuff down that knowing with food. We have been conditioned by society around us to not believe in our own, fullest, potential. We begin to kid ourselves that there are only a few chosen, 'special,' people who can succeed, the rest of us are just destined to watch them from the sofa as though life were one big reality TV show. It is almost as though we have become trapped in a dream and life begins to pass by, full of missed opportunities. This is sacrilege! Life is not reserved for a special few; it is here for all of us to live in our own SPECIAL, unique, way. We all have talents and smiles and love to gift the world. If not us, then who? Do we really want to choose to give our power away to food? Do we not have the urge to choose to taste the whole of life?

It is never too late to fly, never too late to live. It is time to let go now, to let go of looking back. The past is gone and with it our past horrors and pains, we no longer need to hold that. Take a deep breath and choose to let your outrageous vitality emerge now, not tomorrow, not when you reach your 'perfect' shape, not when you finish your degree, not when you get the perfect job or retire. Now, in every moment. Let yourself shine now and your life will change, your dreams may change, your focus may change and shift. If you take one step toward life, life will run to you and embrace you and fill you up before you blink an eye. That is because life and love never left you. It was always there, you just didn't see it because of the food fog that you have been caught within, and there is no need for guilt over that, it's brought you to where you are now and with your new vision you can make a new choice.

If you are afraid and thinking 'I can't let go, I'll fall off the edge' then I promise you that is just an illusion – there are no edges in life, only horizons! If you don't consciously choose life I promise she won't give up on you, she'll call and call and you'll feel the struggle, the pull, and the discomfort of that calling. Make it easy on yourself, give into her now. Jump, leap, skip, and hop into the arms of life. She's ready to catch you, it is impossible to fall because she's everywhere, enveloping you in love, pervading every cell of your being, she was always there, you just didn't see.

Life is vibrant, it is a rainbow, it's bigger than the black and white you've been conditioned to believe exists. The rainbow is beautiful, but not always easy. Life has ups and it has downs. We have to learn to ride those waves, to drink in the color and to TRUST. What is the alternative to that rollercoaster? It's a flat-line, and what is a flat-line? It is dull, and on a hospital monitor a flat-line is death. The ups and downs are life. They are vibrancy.

As Kahlil Gibran writes, in *The Prophet*, about joy and sorrow:

Your joy is your sorrow unmasked.
And the selfsame well from which your laughter rises was oftentimes filled with your tears.
And how else can it be?
The deeper that sorrow carves into your being, the more joy you can contain.
Is not the cup that holds your wine the very cup that was burned in the potter's oven?
And is not the lute that soothes your spirit, the very wood that was hollowed with knives?
When you are joyous, look deep into your heart and you shall find it is only that which has given you sorrow that is giving you joy.
When you are sorrowful look again in your heart, and you shall see that in truth you are weeping for that which has been your delight.

Some of you say, "Joy is greater than sorrow," and others say, "Nay, sorrow is the greater."
But I say unto you, they are inseparable.
Together they come, and when one sits, alone with you at your board, remember that the other is asleep upon your bed.

Verily you are suspended like scales between your sorrow and your joy.
Only when you are empty are you at standstill and balanced.
When the treasure-keeper lifts you to weigh his gold and his silver, needs must your joy or your sorrow rise or fall.

Letting Go Takes Love

To let go does not mean to stop caring; it means I can't do it for someone else.
To let go is not to cut myself off, it's the realization I can't control another.
To let go is not to enable, but allow learning from natural consequences.
To let go is to admit powerlessness, which means the outcome is not in my hands.
To let go is not to try to change or blame another; it's to make the most of myself.
To let go is not to care for, but to care about.
To let go is not to fix, but to be supportive.
To let go is not to judge, but to allow another to be a human being.
To let go is not to be in the middle arranging all the outcomes, but to allow others to affect their destinies.
To let go is not to be protective; it's to permit another to face reality.
To let go is not to deny, but to accept.
To let go is not to nag, scold or argue, but instead to search out

my own shortcomings and correct them.

To let go is not to adjust everything to my desires, but to take each day as it comes and cherish myself in it.

To let go is not to criticize or regulate anybody, but to try to become what I dream I can be.

To let go is not to regret the past, but to grow and live for the future.

To let go is to fear less and love more.

Remember: The time to love is short.

~ Author unknown

Beginning the journey, some self-love tips, quotes and ideas

Take a deep breath. You are so courageous to have stepped into this beautiful journey of loving yourself. Let me honor you for your choice and your commitment and let me assure you that I am here for you, loving you, holding you and encouraging you in every step that you take. It is day one of radically loving yourself. Day one of a lifetime of practicing radical self-love. You are now a self-love revolutionary!

Take time to really praise yourself for beginning. Be proud of yourself. You have chosen to make a commitment to stop waging war on your precious self. Self-loathing and self-hatred is NOT what we were born to feel.

There is a famous true event involving the Dalai Lama that you may have heard before, it is a story that really shines a light on the fact that self-love is something we needn't ever doubt we are worthy of.

In 1990 there was a huge conference in Dharmsala, India. The Dalai Lama, philosophers, psychologists, scientists and meditators were gathered there. Sharon Salzberg, an American long-term meditator and cofounder of the Insight Meditation Society, asked the Dalai Lama a question 'What do you think about self-hatred?' The Dalai Lama replied, 'self-hatred. What is that?' The Dalai Lama did not understand, he had never heard the concept of self-hatred. It took numerous attempts of translation and explanation for him to even begin to know what Sharon was asking. Self-hatred is a mostly Western condition. In Buddhist countries someone not cherishing themselves is quite an unbelievable concept. From the Buddhist point of view there is the belief that every human being has Buddha-nature, has the potential to become fully enlightened. This could equally be applied to the Christian tradition; we all have the potential for Christ Consciousness.

In the Theravada Buddhist tradition there is a lovingkindness meditation that begins with offering lovingkindness to ourselves. The teaching is that lovingkindness for ourselves is a foundation for lovingkindness for others. We can't authentically give to others what we don't have for ourselves.

'You can search throughout the entire universe for someone who is more deserving of your love and affection than you are yourself, and that person is not to be found anywhere. You yourself, as much as anybody in the entire universe deserve your love and affection.'
~ Buddha

The emphasis of loving ourselves is not limited to Buddhism; it is in fact the foundation of any true spiritual understanding.

Breathe in the words of this Lovingkindness meditation:

May I be filled with lovingkindness
May I be well
May I be peaceful and at ease
May I be happy

May you be filled with lovingkindness
May you be well

May you be peaceful and at ease
May you be happy

May all beings be filled with loving kindness
May you be well
May you be peaceful and at ease
May you be happy

In practice it can be easier to break this meditation down into three sections. Here is an idea of how you might wish to practice:

Begin by relaxing into a comfortable posture. Take a few moments to just be with the breath following the in-flow and out-flow. Repeat the following paragraph to yourself, you can read the words with your eyes open until they become easy to remember, then close your eyes and silently repeat the words to yourself:

May I be filled with lovingkindness
May I be well
May I be peaceful and at ease
May I be happy

As you do this meditation, be aware of any areas of tension that you might experience, or resistance that comes up. Be compassionate with yourself. Keep breathing whilst you practice, allow your breath to ease any tensions. Really feel yourself fill up with lovingkindness. Take time after each sentence to fully feel the effects in your body. Keep repeating the sentences over and over again allowing the feelings of lovingkindness to really seep into your body and mind. Be patient with yourself, if difficult feelings of irritation or unkindness/criticism toward yourself surface then acknowledge those feelings with kindness and remember they are just thoughts passing through awareness, come back to the sentences with kindness, friendliness and patience toward yourself.

You might need to practice the first part of this meditation for a number of weeks until allowing lovingkindness for yourself becomes natural and can be done with a sense of ease.

When you feel that you are at ease with lovingkindness for yourself you can move on to the next part of the meditation. Begin your practice with loving kindness for yourself and then, after about 10 minutes, focus on someone in your life that you truly love and care for and who cares for you. Hold them in your heart as you repeat the words below. Really allow your loving feelings to surface as you keep repeating the sentences. Allow your heart to open as wide as possible.

May you be filled with lovingkindness
May you be well
May you be peaceful and at ease
May you be happy

Over time you can continue to add more people into your heart as you do the meditation. Imagine groups of people, neighbors, and communities. Keep expanding your practice as the weeks go by.

As your lovingkindness meditation develops you can include people everywhere, animals and all beings. The meditation will now have three parts, here is the third part:

May the world and all beings be filled with lovingkindness
May the world and all beings be well
May the world and all beings be peaceful and at ease
May the world and all beings be happy

The very final stage of lovingkindness meditation is to include people into your meditation who you might find difficult or annoying and even extend lovingkindness out to those who might be waging war on other countries or criminals. This stage is often the most challenging phase and perhaps you might take years to get to it, and that is fine. Keep in mind that all beings have seeds of goodness within them, no matter what they may have done in life; it is these seeds of goodness that we are watering. We are not condoning their past actions or atrocities.

By doing the lovingkindness meditation we might find over time that our mind seems calmer and we are more connected to our heart and our capacity to love, even in difficult circumstances.

Another way to extend love toward ourselves is to sit silently and repeat a mantra to ourselves. According to Eastern thought/philosophy, a mantra is a word or a phrase that is said to contain spiritual vibration when chanted – the mantra can feed the unconscious mind. A mantra can be a single word such as 'love,' 'tranquility,' or 'peace,' or it can be a sentence or positive affirmation such as 'I deeply and completely love and accept myself,' it can also be a traditional mantra such as my personal favorite, 'Om Namah Shivaya,' which means 'I honor the divinity that resides within me,' – a way of honoring and expressing the divinity that lies at the core of all beings; this is a mantra that can really connect us to our self worth and self-love.

✐ Can you think of some personally comforting and empowering mantras?

Mantras can be relaxing, or can be used to aid relaxation. For example we can follow our breath and silently say 'relax' on the in-breath and 'let go' or 'release' on the out-breath. Mantras feed the unconscious mind so it is important to use a loving and positive mantra. You might find yourself visualizing whilst you repeat a mantra and that's fine! For example, when using the mantra 'peace' this is what comes to me:

The image of a white dove comes to mind, with the image come feelings of relaxation in my body and an opening in the area of my heart. There is a pleasant sensation of warmth throughout my body. In my visualization the dove is landing on the world, on all people, of all colors and creeds and a sense of oneness, unity, interconnection. There is a sense of hope, that world peace could be possible. With this, there is also a sadness around the reality of the present situation in the world, but an intention for change, a belief in change. There is the feeling of being at peace in my life, with my family, in my community. There is the knowing that peace within can impact peace outside. Peace seems to be present as a river of light running through the hearts of all people, connecting us.

Using the mantra 'peace' is not a thought process, there is just a willingness to let go and simply allow feelings and sensations to flow into consciousness, and to notice them within as an impartial observer without attempting to alter them.

🖊 What comes to you when you sit with a chosen mantra? Write about any feelings, images, colors and physical sensations.

The following ideas, prefaced with this love-heart symbol ♥, are included here for you to play with. Here I also include positive affirmations you might want to work with. You might wish to read through all of the ideas and then pick a few that speak to you or that feel like a good first step. In time you might want to come back and build on your self-love practice by including more of the ideas presented here. It is up to you. You might want to take your journal and write about how each pointer makes you feel, or what thoughts, images and emotions come up for you. You might want to leave the section altogether and come back to it at the end of the book or when you feel the time is right. There is no right or wrong way to use these love-tips. Follow your intuition.

♥ Choose to be an ideal parent, or friend to yourself
Nurture yourself as the precious child of the Universe that you are. Be generous, present and loving with yourself. Treat yourself the way you would really love to be treated by others. Treat yourself the way you would treat your own precious child, be your own best friend. If you really looked at how horrible you have been to yourself in the past, in your words, thoughts, deeds you would be shocked. Would you ever dream of treating your own child, or best friend, that way? NO! So now forgive yourself for the past and choose to love, care and be kind to your precious self from now.

Take time to think about how you would love your own precious child or friend, then aim to take concrete steps toward loving yourself in that same way.

An affirmation to try: 'I deserve my own love. I am precious. I love myself unconditionally.'

If you catch yourself being mean to yourself internally with your thoughts then stop, breathe and say something really kind or use the 'I deeply and completely love and accept myself' mantra. This step may well feel challenging, you may be dealing with habits that have lasted a lifetime but we can ALL change, it takes time and patience and self-forgiveness and a whole lot of love but it is completely possible. Know that loving yourself is precious and deserves your time and attention.

'Find the love you seek, by first finding the love within yourself. Learn to rest in that place within you, that is your true home.'
~ Sri Ravi Shankar

♥ Resistance to self-love

'Your task is not to seek for love but merely to seek and find all the barriers within yourself that you have built against it.'
~ Rumi

The resistance you have to loving yourself is probably tied up with 'the voice,' the inner voice of the critic or saboteur. The first step is to acknowledge that this 'voice' is NOT you. Step back and observe it. Usually the inner critic/saboteur is rambling on because it really believes it needs to protect you in some way – if you are successful, happy, free, shining and loving yourself then it believes this means danger. The critic/saboteur believes that shining your light may mean you have to be more or do more, so it attempts to stop you by saying you are not worthy, it would be selfish to love yourself, who are you to think you can be so much?

Geneen Roth speaks about 'The Voice' in her book, *Women, Food and God*. She writes:

The Voice usurps your strength, passion and energy and then turns them against you...leaves you feeling defeated and weak, which then leaves you susceptible to latching on to the next quick fix or miracle cure. The Voice is merciless, ravaging, life destroying. The Voice makes you feel so weak, so paralyzed, so incompetent that you wouldn't dare question its authority.

Your first step is to recognize this critical, sabotaging voice/thoughts are not who you are. Byron Katie says, 'I love my thoughts. I'm just not tempted to believe them.' When you realize you are hearing this negative inner talk, STOP, BREATHE and relax. Congratulate yourself for disengaging and then say, 'Even though I feel_____ or even though I think_____ I deeply and completely love and accept myself.' Love is SO POWERFUL. Love yourself, replace those critical thoughts with positive ones and slowly the thoughts will change over time. For some ideas of positive affirmations you can look at the website www.youcanhealyourlife.com or check out any books by Louise Hay, she is queen of positive affirmations.

No more beating yourself up. The resistance you feel really isn't YOU. Keep loving yourself, love the resistance, love the journey.

♥ Take breath stops

Remember to STOP and BREATHE during the day. Doing this helps to take us out of our heads and into our hearts. It allows for communication between the head and heart, it allows us to hear our needs and feel our feelings. Follow your breathing especially at times when everything seems like 'too much.' Imagine love entering with each in-breath and anxiety leaving with each exhale. Experiment with setting your phone so that it buzzes every hour; this can be really helpful to bring you back into a state of awareness and acts as a prompt to remind you to breathe deeply, to relax your shoulders, to relax the tensions in your body and mind. What do you notice when you take time to breathe deeply?

'I breathe in love and life and I am relaxed.'

♥ Slow down

Allow yourself to stop rushing. Feel the moment without always thinking ahead. This moment is a gift, you won't have it again. Life is not a race to the finish line, enjoy the journey.

'I slow down and cherish the moment.'

Sit down for ten minutes and really taste a cup of herbal tea or a fresh juice. Feel the warmth of the mug in your hands and drink in the comfort of the hot liquid. Allow the moment to nurture you. The universe is in that mug of tea – the sun, rain, soil, plants, the farm workers and the shop assistants who sold it to you. The chain of life is mesmerizing.

'I relax and take time to taste life.'

♥ Feed your mind
Switch off the mindless TV and stop watching gruesome, frightening or miserable programs that don't feel good. Allow your mind to be watered with positive images.

'I choose to allow positive images to enter my vision.'

♥ Allow yourself to play
You are a child of the universe, allow yourself to experience the beauty of play, pleasure and laughter.

'I allow myself to feel joyful and happy.'

Explore what this means to you. Can you allow yourself to play and be happy? It took me a while to learn to allow myself to really experience joy. For years I believed I wasn't worthy of joy, my grandparents had been through a terrible time in world war two and for some reason I had decided that because of their painful past I didn't have the right to express joy. It wasn't until a powerful moment during the counseling course I was studying when I truly felt that my grandparents wanted me to be the happiest person I could be, and to express it out into the world. They wanted me to know that it was my gift to be happy and playful, it wasn't disrespectful at all. In fact NOT playing and enjoying my freedom was disrespectful, it was what they had pushed for, my freedom!

Have a look at your limiting beliefs about play. What blocks does your critic or saboteur, 'the voice' put up? Go forwards with a big heart and love and enjoy this precious life.

What could you today that you would really enjoy? Could you take a salsa dancing class? Or just dance around in your favorite dress? Would you really like to learn to sew, craft or paint? How about swimming for fun and not for fitness? Would you love to go out for lunch with a friend or play with your dog outside? What would fill your soul?

Experiment with different forms of creativity. Perhaps you could investigate some of the really interesting adult, mosaic and pattern coloring books, these can be challenging but taking the time to just color, without criticism or expectation of results, can also help the mind to become expansive and free from thought.

♥ The power of touch and pampering
Take time to pamper your precious body. Soak in a bath, don't rush your shower, rub lotion into your dry skin, wrap yourself in a soft blanket and snuggle up in a comfortable spot.

'I lovingly take care of my precious body. I give myself permission to take gentle care of myself.'

Ask for a hug. Treat yourself to a massage. Ask your lover to touch you in exactly the way you would most like.

'I allow and enjoy the healing power of touch.'

It is often said that your body is your temple, your precious vehicle here on earth. It's time to really treat your body well, to love it, to nourish it, to care for it. You can start now. Notice any resistance but still start now. As you care for your body say loving things to yourself, talk to yourself gently. If you are finding it really difficult then say, 'I am willing to learn to love and care for my precious body, I am willing and I begin to take action now.'

Stop waiting for a special occasion to wear the clothes that make you feel good, or to express yourself through your clothes. Life is your special occasion and you are worthy of feeling like a Goddess each day.

'I am worthy of feeling good about what I wear whatever the occasion. I choose to dress myself in ways that truly express the wonder of me.'

♥ The glorious art of receiving

Many women that I have worked with say that they find it almost impossible to receive anything from anyone – compliments, gifts, offers of help, money etc. It is often the case that they believe that they just don't deserve anything. Slowly you can begin to learn that life is in a natural, continual flow of giving and receiving. Slowly you can learn that you don't just have to give, give, give, you are worthy of receiving too. The Universe likes to be in a constant flow – we breathe out carbon dioxide which plants and trees lovingly use and provide us with much needed oxygen in return. Begin by learning how to receive compliments with grace. Allow yourself to truly receive what people offer you. Smile and say 'thank you' instead of brushing off the gift that is being offered to you. Open your heart to the compliment, let it fill you up, allow it to nourish your beautiful soul.

♥ Letting go of comparisons

You are unique, fall in love with that uniqueness. No one

else has your eyes, your fingers or your way of loving. We are all equally unique. Incessant comparison breeds depression and despair. Let go and fall into the pillow of self-love, it will allow you to love others more fully in their uniqueness too.

'I love my uniqueness and I love and honor the uniqueness of others.'

When you let go of comparisons do you feel freer? More free to be yourself?

Do you find that you are spending a lot of time comparing yourself negatively to everyone? Magazines are often especially difficult for many women; they are filled with perfectly airbrushed images that look out at us. Our own precious, beautiful bodies may seem so different in comparison and we can easily feel as though we could never reach that level of beauty. When we think like this it is because we are forgetting our own unique awesomeness. No, we may well not look like the images we see, however, no one will ever look like you either. We need to learn, to rejoice in ourselves and celebrate our preciousness. Sometimes I still fall into the comparison trap but these days I don't buy those magazines or look at those images, instead I take time to nourish my own uniqueness and find my own place in this wonderful world. I enjoy celebrating the uniqueness of my friends and family. It's wonderful that we all have our own particular gorgeous body to wear in the world.

Stop making jokes at your own expense, or at the expense of others. Put-downs are unpleasant, they don't feed the soul and they can wound in a way we may not be aware of. Find positive things to say about yourself and others.

'I choose to find, and highlight, the positive in myself and others.'

Make a list today of all the things that are great about you. Can you mention some of these things when you are with other people rather than putting yourself down? We find it so easy to make ourselves small, but today we need to start a habit of allowing ourselves to shine out and be LARGE. There really is no need to play small. Shine your light into the world!

Trying to impress others is a waste of your energy. Love only wants you to be true to yourself, to live your best life in your own way. Be congruent with who you really are, that is truly impressive and will inspire others too.

'I am congruent with my true self.'

♥ Stop giving out well-meaning advice to others
Concentrate on loving them as they are. This will allow you to love yourself more as you are. Listen with a wide-open heart and be gentle when you speak.

'I love others the way I would like to be loved and I listen fully without needing to give advice.'

♥ Stop the constant analysis
Take time to fall in love with the mystery of life. Let go of analyzing conversations and situations. Sometimes we just don't know why things happen, why people say things or what things may mean. Concentrate on your own clarity of speech, be loving in your actions and then step away.

'Life is a fabulous mystery.'

Love is like a well that can never dry out. It can be used but never used up, the supply is endless. Drink it in daily, let it nourish you and infuse every situation.

'I allow love to continually flow to me and through me.'

♥ Watch what you make things mean

Sometimes people will attach their own meanings to what you say or do – you may say 'no' and they might make that mean something about them or you, when all you have said is 'no.' We need to stop attaching our own meanings to what people say and instead just hear their words. A teacher on a course I was doing once said, 'if you saw someone you knew walking down the street and you called out and said hello but they didn't answer and carried on walking what would you think?' Would you make that mean the person didn't like you? Was ignoring you? Was angry with you for something? Or would you think they just didn't hear you? That they were late for something? Or could you just think 'oh' and carry on walking without making it mean anything? Our minds can create such stories. It really is time to stop the analysis, to be aware of what the mind is telling us and to let go. Just let go and LOVE.

See and feel the Divine in your own eyes and in the eyes of others. Offer a prayer of recognition when you connect with other people. Whisper the word Namaste to yourself.

Namaste translates as: 'I honor the place in you where the entire universe resides. I honor the place in you of love, of truth, of peace and of light, and when you are in that place in you and I am in that place in me, there is only one of us.'

'Om Namah Shivaya' – 'I honor the Divinity that resides within me' – honor that in others too.

Feel the interconnection between all beings. We are all manifested from the un-manifest; we are all pieces of the Divine experiencing life. See Divinity in the eyes of every person you meet and in your own self too. Love the Divine in you and in all.

'I see Divinity in the eyes of all beings and I see it in my own self. Love is the glue that holds us all together.'

♥ Love for yourself as a doorway
Unconditional love for yourself opens the doorway to authentic love for others. If we could all develop unconditional love for ourselves then world peace really would be inevitable. It takes courage to participate in changing yourself and loving yourself, but in this way you impact the world and become a beacon for love and a teacher for others.

Being loving toward ourselves helps us to be more loving toward others. Communicating kindly with ourselves can have a knock on impact for the way we communicate with others. For more tips on loving communication visit the website www.nonviolentcommunication.com. They have lots of free resources available.

♥ Remember not to believe everything you think
Thoughts are just thoughts, they are not who you are, observe them and then remember to say, 'even though I feel _____ I deeply and completely love and accept myself.' Check out The Work of Byron Katie at http://www.thework.com/index.php. She uses four questions to get us to examine our beliefs:

1. Is it true?
2. Can you absolutely know that it's true?
3. How do you react, what happens, when you believe that thought?
4. Who would you be without the thought?

Painful thoughts are often attempting to keep us small, in the belief they will keep us safe. Shining in the world isn't dangerous, it is wonderful and beautiful.

If you have past, painful memories coming up then I would

urge you to go and explore counseling, in order to get those past experiences out of your head. You can search for registered professional counselors at the British Association for Counseling and Psychotherapy: http://www.itsgoodtotalk. org.uk/therapists.

'The world we have created is a product of our thinking. It cannot be changed without changing our thinking.'
~ Albert Einstein

It is time to begin changing our thoughts daily, to loving, self-loving thoughts. Envisage what your life would be like now if you continued to choose to love yourself daily.

♥ Unconditional Love

'Loving people doesn't mean you have to enjoy their company, want to see more of them, or even respect their values. It means you're willing to keep your heart open to them, show them compassion and accept them for who they are.'
~ Marci Shimoff

For me, 'I love you unconditionally' doesn't mean that I agree with you, like you or even approve of you. I don't expect you to agree with me, like me or approve of me either. I love you anyway, warts and all, in your humanness, in your wholeness, as a saint and a sinner. I may not remember your birthday or give you what you want or need, but I do love you.

Rambunctious resources for the exploration of self-love

♥ Lisa Clark. *Sassy. The go-for-it girl's guide to becoming mistress of your destiny.*

♥ Mimi Shannon's wonderful website:
http://www.meloveletters.com

♥ A great website with self-compassion tests:
http://www.self-compassion.org

♥ Tara Brach. *Radical Acceptance. Embracing your life with the heart of a Buddha.*

♥ Kim McMillen. *When I loved myself enough.*

♥ Regena Thomashauer. *Mama Gena's school of womanly arts. Using the power of pleasure to have your way with the world.*

♥ Cheryl Richardson. *The art of extreme self care.*

Chapter 6

You were born to sparkle and to shine

The use of food can often represent an unconscious way of being noticed; if we really over-ate continuously we would be noticed for physically taking up space. However, we can also make the choice and give ourselves permission to shine and sparkle and take up space in this world through loving ourselves first, rather than turning to food first. If you lavish love on yourself your inner sparkle will shine out. The pain of self-loathing and inner critical-self talk takes up space, if we replace it with the voice of love and empowerment we will feel freer, and more than this, it gives permission for the women around us to shine. We need to break the chains that bind us to old beliefs and old patterns.

We were not created to hide our talents and our particular flavor of sparkle. Your soul knows that, you know that. You are allowed to take up space, physically and with your smile and that inner sparkle that comes from love.

✐ Journal about how you feel when you read about giving yourself permission to shine. Can you do that or are you blocked by thoughts, which tell you this is selfish or narcissistic? Take time to explore these feelings and thoughts, see if you can give yourself the permission you need to begin to thrive and shine.

Think about all the time and energy that goes into negative self-talk. Have you ever been in the middle of a conversation with a dear friend but actually you're not really listening because you are obsessing about the size of your thighs or stomach? This is NOT an opportunity for you to be critical toward yourself or judgmental, just notice your inner experience, be aware. Think about how it might be without the obsession, if you just woke up every day and decided to shine your awesomeness instead? You could be more present to your own needs as well as the needs of others. Hating on our precious selves is exhausting, it takes up time and energy and can lead us to depression. Imagine what we could be doing with that time and energy; imagine how fantastic we could make life. We have that power within us right now.

You have to give yourself the unconditional love that you seek from others. For many years I was the 'good-girl-pleaser,' giving was enjoyable but beneath all of that I wanted to be loved too. Many of my friendships and relationships were unhealthy, I didn't love myself in the slightest, I didn't know I was allowed to love myself. I thought that I was only supposed to give love. On some level I resented that, but I thought resentment was bad so I ate to squash it all down – which meant I felt worse and I would attempt to give more and the cycle just went on. When I did begin to take care of myself, give my needs attention and love myself, people left my life. This was a good thing on some levels but on others it was trauma, especially when one friend left my life, someone who I really trusted and really thought would support me in my quest to love myself. After-all, I was still giving love, just in a healthier way and I had boundaries. My essence of love had not changed.

My personal journey toward self-love included a four-year stint of not being in a romantic relationship. I read, wrote, learned, had therapy, went on courses, studied and loved myself. When I least expected it I met Chris, who is now my husband. Our love grows all the time and it's not always pretty, but it is honest and true. It may sound like a cliché but love really is like a rose – the radiantly beautiful blooms, the great times, that we appreciate stay for a short while before they die off, then there are less picturesque times but the love remains in other forms, ready for another bloom. Love can be thorny; there can be periods of quiet and reflection and then re-growth. Most of all, the manure, the mulch, the dirt, the challenging stuff – that feeds the rose, if we can work through it with love and patience and openness it becomes the energy that powers us forwards. Those 'dark' shadowy, manure, places are as important as the light, bright, blooms, they make up part of the whole. We cannot deny the whole. It can be embraced and that's what makes life so beautiful.

Just let go of your tight grip on the obsession of self-hating-talk. Let it go. At first it can feel as though you are falling into an abyss with no life-line, but self-love is there to catch you. Self-love is your natural state. It can feel frightening. You may feel that if you let go and stop hating yourself you might eat yourself to death from gaining so much weight, or whatever. Those thoughts can be terrifying. They are just thoughts.

When you start to love yourself you begin to realize that there is nothing stopping you from reaching your dreams, nothing stopping you from going travelling, changing jobs, moving location or ending destructive friendships and relationships. Yet this knowledge is also terrifying. There is nothing stopping you from life! You begin to realize that it is time to take responsibility for living life and not hiding from it, you realize that you need to take action steps. You are allowed to be happy. Self-hate has probably been sabotaging your sparkle for so long that when it begins to diminish and self-love begins to burst forth you may not know quite what to do.

Take one step at a time. Go slow. My journey began with getting help and asking for support, I had therapy and allowed myself to begin doing things I wanted to do, slowly. More than once daily I reminded myself that the journey of a thousand miles begins with a single step. I wasn't going to allow self-hate to hold me back. Remember that self-loathing is often just a veil for a deeper feeling and a deeper need (we will look at feelings and needs later). We can allow these feelings and needs to surface into our awareness without being hard on ourselves. We can find safe friendships and groups where we can share our stories and hence release them with no judgments.

🖉 If you really loved yourself:

- How would you talk to yourself?
- What would you wear?
- What would you do for relaxation?
- What would you do for pleasure?
- What events would you go to?
- What events would you say 'no' to?
- What would you choose to eat and drink?
- What would your friends be like?
- What hobbies would you try?
- How would you make love?
- How would you walk?
- How would you treat yourself?
- How would you play?
- How would you move your body?
- How would you begin your day?
- What areas of your life would you lovingly change?
- How much sleep would you get?
- What TV shows would you watch?
- What dreams would you take steps towards?

That is just a moment away, a choice away. What would it take for you to decide to love yourself? Do you need to forgive yourself your past in order to move on? Do it. You are not a 'bad' person. You're a whole person; self-love is a gift you are allowed to give to yourself.

🖉 Make a list of things you value in yourself. Imagine how your best friend or your soul would describe you. Concentrate on being willing to change your inner dialogue.

There is nothing wrong with you my sweet, sweet, precious soul-sister. There is so, so much right with you. You are not 'bad,' your problems with food are not wrong, they do not make you less deserving of life or happiness. You are a beautiful woman, sacred and soulful. Just wake up from the dream of feeling so wrong. Falling in love with yourself is not something that can wait. You deserve it now. You are already love. At your core you know that you are deserving, that you can be kind to yourself and that it is vital.

Cultural conditioning, your up-bringing, society, media, this influences you but it doesn't control you. Deep down you know that it is not 'bad' to feel great about yourself, it is not bad to celebrate who you are. You do not need to use food any more to stuff down your feelings, your needs, and your urge to shine. Allow your True Essence to unfold within your precious heart and know that who you are at your core is enough, in fact it is so great and amazing that it wants to burst forth and not be squashed down with food anymore – but even if you continue to use food for the rest of your life as a coping mechanism then love yourself anyway, break the chain of negative self-talk that pierces your soul. Love yourself. Do it now.

It is important to build, maintain and strengthen your self-love muscle as a daily practice. You may not always feel self-loving but it is still possible to practice loving yourself on a daily basis. Envisage your self-love nurturer as a part of you, this nurturer loves you unconditionally, no matter what you say or do. They are always there for you, never critical, never harsh. Always listening and supportive and there to help you to explore your feelings deeply and safely. The nurturer is part of your Divine Nature.

We all have a choice. Our self-abuse can stop here. The loathing and the criticism can stop. We do not have to beat up on ourselves just because we hear women all around us doing it. We have to break the chain, for ourselves and for future generations of women. Nurture yourself with great care. Be as nice to yourself as you can be. Honor the Divinity within you, know that the Goddess is there and she won't let you down. You are precious and loved. When the critical voices begin, hold yourself tighter and say nice things to yourself. Take time for your life. Who says it isn't ok to take care of your precious self? Let other people say what you like, what they think is none of your business and it's sad if they are so bitter and critical, it's a reflection of their own inner critic. By modeling self-love you are liberating many women from their self-imposed prisons.

Be prepared for the voice of criticism to show up when things get good!

Once you have become fairly used to loving yourself you might find that your use of food for comfort died right down. Suddenly you may become aware that you feel freer, happier, more empowered, and more joyful. This is when you need to be really aware of your inner voice and criticism. It is likely that the saboteur will show up now and urge you toward food – because it fears that you are becoming 'too much,' 'too bright.' The critic will try to convince you that it is not ok to feel good about yourself. This is when you need to use the nurturing voice of self-love. You are allowed to shine, to be awesome, to feel attractive and not apologize for your very existence.

We have to break the chain for women. It is madness to think that there is only one acceptable body shape. It is madness to believe that we are not allowed to feel the full spectrum of emotions and to have needs. We need to start working toward shining and not using food to dim our own light. We are all whole pieces of Divinity. There is a Goddess within. We have no need to measure up to anyone else. Go within, what is your True Nature walking you toward? Follow that. Find your own flavor in this world, your own path. Food is our fuel, our medicine and it can be our celebration, but it has no power other than what we give it. The power within us is our Divinity embodied. All of us will have our own sparkle. It might be strong, or exuberant, quiet or loud, vibrant, rich, soft. Flow with it and life will become richer.

'Be strong then, and enter into your own body; there you have a solid place for your own feet.'

~ Kabir

This quote speaks of spiritual embodiment. My wish for you is not to be slim, or curvy, or weigh a certain weight. My wish for you is to see and honor the Divinity that resides within you and to find peace with your awesome power and hence with food. My wish is that you shine uniquely as you.

Oriah Mountain Dreamer, in *The Dance*, writes:

When we believe that we are by our very nature deeply flawed – self-indulgent, selfish, judgmental, sinful – our efforts to fulfill our soul's longing to live fully become efforts to control, chastise, reshape, improve, and change ourselves. Believing we are by nature lazy and unworthy, we believe we will not change, will not become the people we want to be unless we are pushed or forced by suffering to do so. Given this belief, we use methods that do not cultivate mercy and compassion for ourselves but rather foster a hardness toward our own suffering and the suffering of those who are failing to curb or rise above their basic nature.

When we judge like that we cannot be all that we are. Our True Nature is so much more than most of us are willing to accept. Loving ourselves without reservations opens the gateway for us to love. To love deeply. We cannot bash ourselves into shape – it doesn't work. Love yourself. Do it now. Do it deeply.

Real compassion can help you shine

We've been discussing self-love as a bedrock, a foundation, for letting go of emotional eating. Having compassion for ourselves and the mistakes we make is a huge part of this self-love and self-care process. However, REAL compassion isn't all nicey-nicey, roses down the garden path, pink, sparkly yumminess. NO. Sometimes real compassion can feel painful because it pushes on our self-imposed boundaries, it isn't politically correct and it doesn't let us get away with self-harm, it doesn't massage the ego. The term 'idiot compassion' was coined by a Buddhist teacher named Chogyam Trungpa Rinpoche who said:

> Idiot compassion is the highly conceptualized idea that you want to do good... Of course, [according to the mahayana teachings of Buddhism] you should do everything for everybody; there is no selection involved at all. But that doesn't mean to say that you have to be gentle all the time. Your gentleness should have heart, strength. In order that your compassion doesn't become idiot compassion, you have to use your intelligence. Otherwise, there could be self-indulgence of thinking that you are creating a compassionate situation when in fact you are feeding the other person's aggression. If you go to a shop and the shopkeeper cheats you and you go back and let him cheat you again, that doesn't seem to be a very healthy thing to do for others.

For example, if you were in a relationship where there was violence, either emotional aggression or physical hitting, it would not be compassionate to stay in that situation simply because you loved the person and didn't want to hurt their feelings by leaving. Actually leaving the relationship would be a difficult thing to do but it would be the compassionate choice, for you and the other person. Pema Chodron writes of this situation:

> It's the compassionate thing to do for yourself, because you're part of that dynamic, and before you always stayed. So now you're going to do something frightening, groundless, and

quite different. But it's the compassionate thing to do for yourself, rather than stay in a demeaning, destructive, abusive relationship. And it's the most compassionate thing you can do for them too. They will certainly not thank you for it, and they will certainly not be glad. They'll go through a lot. But if there's any chance for them to wake up or start to work on their side of the problem, their abusive behavior or whatever it might be, that's the only chance, is for you to actually draw the line and get out of there.

In terms of food and eating; idiot compassion, ego-massaging compassion, would tell you that it is ok to eat the whole box of chocolates because you love chocolates and to be kind to yourself you must give yourself exactly what you wish, right? No Way! Real compassion is very wise. It is wisdom compassion. Wise/real compassion is caring but not always sweet. Wise compassion would not say it was OK to eat the whole box of chocolates. Wise compassion might say, 'have one chocolate and savor the taste of it and have a few nuts too to help balance your blood sugar and prevent you binging the whole box of chocolates,' or, wise compassion would assess the situation and say, 'you know what, you are really emotional today so it is best to stay away from the chocolates. Let's sit down quietly for a moment and tune in to what you really need right now.' Wise, real, compassion does not let us get away with self-harming behaviors. Of course, if we have already eaten the whole box of chocolates wise compassion does not beat us up over it and criticize us mercilessly either, wise compassion might say something like 'you've made a mistake, let's learn from this so that next time you listen to your real needs before you binge eat.'

We will be looking at watching our thoughts and allowing our feelings and needs later; wise compassion always sees the bigger picture and takes into account the real issues. Self-love and compassion are fierce in the sense that they fiercely love you with wisdom. Self-love and wise compassion would not say, 'you've had a hard day honey so let's sit down and eat a tub of ice-cream to soothe ourselves.' NO. Wise compassion might say, 'you've had a hard day honey, let's have a hot bath or a walk, or let's call a friend or read a nurturing book.' Tune into your wise self, it is always there, inextricably linked into the very fabric of your being. Practice wise compassion; love yourself with a fierce wisdom.

🖉 Journal about how you could be more wisely compassionate with yourself. Take time to also journal about how 'idiot compassion' may have sabotaged your growth and happiness in the past.

Chapter 7

Being aware of thoughts

Imagine yourself standing on the bank of a river; the rushing water represents your thoughts. You watch these thoughts go by, some are empowering, e.g. 'what a beautiful day,' 'I am so excited about finishing that project,' 'I am looking forward to Katie coming over for lunch,' some are disempowering, e.g. 'it's awful being stuck inside when the sun is out,' 'this project is taking ages and is so draining,' 'I can't cope with Katie coming for lunch, I hate eating with people.'

Notice this stream of thoughts without judgment. Just notice, be interested. Often there is an 'inner critic' or saboteur shouting inside, 'you're fat, ugly, lazy, going nowhere, doing it all wrong, a loser, you can't change, you'll never do it right.' This critic drowns out the gentle, kind and loving voice which whispers, 'you are enough, you are loved, you are doing so well, I love you.'

Stand back and observe all of these thoughts. You are on the river bank watching them all flow by. This is so empowering and a great step – you are not your thoughts – you are the observer, the witness, the awareness itself. You watch the thoughts go by. You can dis-identify from the thoughts. Too often we fall into the river and get swept away, we become so stressed and entangled in the thoughts that we believe they are real and that in some way we are the thoughts. The stress of listening to all this inner criticism can lead to eating, often unconsciously, as a way to cope.

Sometimes the thoughts are rapid and sometimes they are slow and gentle. If we can remain as the impartial observer, the blissful awareness, and not believe them then we are making a great step toward peace and we will be less likely to unconsciously reach for food as a coping mechanism.

🖉 Take 10 minutes to sit and write down the stream of thoughts passing through your mind. Notice how the thoughts change and pass from moment to moment. Notice that you are observing those thoughts. Write about the experience, does it feel empowering to create a gap between who you are and your thinking?

Another way to look at thoughts is to imagine them as a storm. Now, you probably know that the centre of the storm, the eye, is peaceful and calm? We need to learn to stand at the centre of the storm and watch the thoughts rage around us, knowing we are safe and peaceful as the observer in the centre. In fact we are the 'I' at the centre of the thought storm. The observer, the 'I', our True Nature is always calm, never tangled in the thoughts. It's just that we forget, we latch onto a thought and believe it is us! We try to run from the storm to escape it and usually we run for food, which actually pushes us deeper into the storms of thought and criticism.

When you begin to notice the inner unrest, pause and breathe, create a gap between you as the observer and the thoughts that arise. You are not a slave to your thinking mind. Be curious with your thoughts, notice how you react. Noticing is the first step.

Challenge your thinking

Now that you have begun to observe your thinking, (which is actually a key aspect of meditation, observing without judgment or reaction and bringing yourself back to the centre of the storm, to the river bank, to the peaceful calm of 'I'), you can become more curious and begin practicing, taking a pause and choosing empowering thoughts, so that that quiet voice of calm becomes louder. When there is a gap, a space for breath, there is also a space for healing, for choosing a more loving way to deal with any issues. You might find that you can choose not to eat and instead experiment with other self-soothing strategies (which we will look at later).

All or nothing thinking or black and white thoughts. These are extreme thoughts, which look a little something like this:

> I will never be able to stop comfort eating;
> I am giving up chocolate forever;
> I should go to the gym every day;
> I am worthless;
> I cannot cope with life;
> When I stop comfort eating I can be happy;
> Eating is my only comfort and my only joy.

✎ What are your most common extreme thoughts? Take time to also write out some alternative, more empowering, thoughts.

As mentioned earlier, nothing is black and white. We tend to catergorize our thoughts and lives into boxes. Good v Bad, Right v Wrong, but life is not like that. Extreme thoughts are harsh and destructive and do not lead to healing. We can question these thoughts. Ask yourself, 'is this thought really true?' 'Does this kind of thinking make me feel happy or miserable?,' 'can I think about this in a more positive way?' 'Would it be more helpful to observe my thinking and choose a new thought?' Ask yourself whether you would like to think in a new way, give yourself permission to think in a new, more loving, way. Can you see how you are beating yourself up with your words?

✎ Are the people in your life also black and white thinkers? Do you find yourself taking on their negative thoughts? Could you bring yourself to be positive around them or does your relationship thrive on the drama and negativity? Gently take a look at that. Investigate yourself, could you make small changes in the way you communicate?

Many conversations between women center around weight loss, feeling fat, needing to shed weight, not being good enough. The more aware you become of your inner self talk, the more aware you will become of the conversations around you. There are so many more amazing conversations that we could be having. You have the power to begin to change the way you speak with your female friends. This can be done gently and courageously, e.g. 'do you think we might stay away from talking about dieting today?' 'I'd really rather talk about this amazing art exhibition that I saw yesterday rather than dwell on the weight loss stuff again.' It may well be a slow process but when you begin to change your thoughts you can begin to change your conversations too. You can choose to put your attention onto positive topics, empowering and interesting topics!

Read this quote carefully, let it sink in, let it empower you. Can you see that life is not black and white? Can you see that you are not a 'bad person' because you emotionally overeat at times? Can you have compassion for yourself? Compassion is vital for change. The voice of self-hate can be quietened with the voice of self-love and self-compassion. Do you dare to let go of your negative, destructive, thoughts and live?

I am not here to become an acceptable person, I am here to accept the person I am.

It may be true that you make sacrifices, but that doesn't make you good, it just means that you make sacrifices.

It may be true that you are accepting but that doesn't make you good, it means that you are accepting.

It may be true that you are responsible but that doesn't make you good, it means you are responsible.

It may be true that you meditate, but that doesn't make you good, it just means you meditate.

We label these behaviors good and then continue to do them in order to support self-hate. Perhaps doing in order to be good is what keeps you from realizing that you are already good.

It may be true that you gossip, but that doesn't make you bad, it just means you gossip.

It may be true that you tell lies, but that doesn't make you bad, it just means you tell lies.

It may be true that you are impatient, but that doesn't make you bad, it just means you are impatient.

It may be true that you are sarcastic, but that doesn't make you bad, it just means you are sarcastic.

We label these behaviors as bad and then continue to do them in order to support self-hate. Believing that what you do determines who you are could be the real reason for continuing the behaviors.

It's a lose/lose game with self-hate.

If I feel good I have to pay the price because it's not really okay to feel good.

If I feel bad I have to pay the price because it's not really okay to feel bad.

The only way out of this life of suffering is through the doorway of compassion. 'But how do I find the doorway?' You can't find it because you are it. The moment there is nothing left of you but compassion, you ARE the doorway. The door is open and you are free.

~ Cheri Huber, *There is nothing wrong with you – Going beyond self-hate, a compassionate process for learning to accept yourself exactly as you are.*

Loving thoughts

We've already looked deeply into self-love. It is important to practice these loving ways of thinking until they become natural and easy.

🖋 Here are a few examples of loving thoughts, see if you can think of a few that feel personally nourishing to you:

I deeply and completely love and accept myself;

I can learn something from this;

I now see how I can do things differently;

I am safe; I now do something to take care of myself;

I appreciate myself;

I am loved;

Everything I need to know is revealed to me;

I can comfort myself with love.

Each time you hear the negative thoughts say STOP (either silently in your mind, or out loud!) and then repeat something loving to yourself like: 'I deeply and completely love and accept myself,' 'I am willing to change,' 'I am willing to learn to love myself.' No more self blame. Be fearlessly loving with your thoughts. Remember you are not your thoughts, don't let them bully you.

Accepting and loving our wholeness

We are whole, beautiful beings but all too often we deny what makes us, us; we deny our wholeness. As an example from my own life: For years I took on the narrow persona of 'The Good Girl.' I believed that I was only loveable if I was good, helpful, giving, quiet, hardworking and a pleaser. The problem with that approach to life was that I became completely exhausted, shattered and shut down to the beauty of my broad spectrum of gifts. My wish to love and please others was so strong that I almost forgot that I even existed. It took a painful relationship breakdown and a serious illness to wake me, and shake me up, to push me into embracing my self-love journey.

In life we tend to push down the darker 'shadow' parts, labeling them as 'bad' rather than just accepting them as part of being human. Or, we focus on them thinking that we are rotten to the core, all the while denying our light aspects. It is important to love what we believe is unlovable in ourselves. The problem is that by denying and pushing our so-called unlovable parts away, we often unconsciously act out from them. We self-sabotage, judge others and, in general, end up feeling awful about ourselves.

What's really interesting is, that quite often, what annoys us about another person is actually what most annoys us about ourselves, but because we have denied it, we see it in everyone else. The good news is that it works the other way around as well: what we admire about another person is actually what exists within us too, but we haven't yet owned.

Meredith Brooks and Alanis Morrisette both sang, 'I'm a Bitch.' The lyrics speak of honoring our wholeness (here's an excerpt from the chorus):

I'm a bitch, I'm a lover
I'm a child, I'm a mother
I'm a sinner, I'm a saint
I do not feel ashamed
I'm your hell, I'm your dream
I'm nothing in between
You know you wouldn't want it any other way

We also split emotions into 'bad' and 'good' but emotions are as they are, neither good nor bad. In the light of non-judgmental awareness things are as they are, neither better, nor worse. Anger, joy, jealousy, happiness – these emotions are equally valid, all are important. So have compassion for your wholeness, for your humanness. Be a witness to life and not the victim. Self-love is definitely a daily journey and certainly not a destination. Integrating all of our 'denied parts' can be difficult and emotional. We need to seek out support. This help can come from many sources such as therapists, books, courses and groups. Look into the support that you feel would be most lovingly beneficial to your on your journey.

Often when we begin our self-love journey we have resistance to loving our whole self. That resistance is most often tied to 'the voice,' the inner voice of the critic or saboteur. A first big step is to acknowledge that this 'voice' is NOT you. Sit back and observe it. Usually the inner critic/saboteur is rambling on because it really believes its job is to protect you in some way. For some of us, our inner critic believes that if we are successful, happy, free, shining and loving ourselves, we are in danger. The critic/saboteur may also believe that shining your light could mean you have to be more or do more, so it attempts to stop you by saying you are not worthy, or selfish, or even arrogant to think you are big and can make a difference.

The stories that our minds tell us are endless, there we find struggle – we believe we would be happy in a different body, house or country, a different relationship. Or we think that every-thing would be perfect if we had more money and the right car and pair of shoes. The mind spins out all these stories and we get hooked into them believing that they are real and forgetting that these are just thoughts. When we get carried away believing these stories we miss out on real life – the tiny flower growing out of the crack in the pavement on our walk to the bus stop, the warmth and touch of a friends hug, the silence of a still morning. We miss out on life. Instead we walk along worrying and strug-gling and ending up in the kitchen, eating. Just stop, pause, breathe, be here now, be present in the moment. Feel your feet on the floor. No story. Let the mental chatter continue without hooking into it, wake up to the perfect, present, eternal moment.

We are whole human beings. Everyone has internal rubbish and pain. The difference is, when we begin to heal, when we become authentic we decide not to put chocolate on top of our rubbish in an attempt to make it seem sweeter. We begin to stop reacting from our unconscious mind, from our shadows. Yes, sometimes we trip, we fall back into old patterns, we make mistakes and hurt ourselves or do something that someone else feels hurt by. In these times we must find forgiveness for ourselves. We can be unashamedly who we are and in that we recognize that we do our best in each moment to be the best of our abilities. It is an ongoing journey, but observing our thoughts means we become more able to act and speak from a place of peace and not unconsciousness.

✐ How do you feel about being 'whole,' can you accept all of who you are? What have you labeled as 'bad' and what do you cherish as 'good?'

Rambunctious resources for the exploration of thoughts

- ♥ The work of Byron Katie.
  http://www.thework.com/index.php
- ♥ Cheri Huber. *There is nothing wrong with you. Going beyond self-hate. A compassionate process for learning to accept yourself exactly as you are.*
- ♥ Louise Hay. *You can heal your life.*
- ♥ Debbie Ford. *The dark side of the light chasers. Reclaiming your power, creativity, brilliance, and dreams.*
- ♥ Debbie Ford. *Why good people do bad things. How to stop being your own worst enemy.*

Chapter 8

Take action for change

We have just had a look at thoughts and watching them and replacing them with other thoughts. This is all very important work, but there comes a point when we have to make concrete, out in the world, changes to the way we operate.

As humans we are creatures of habit, we like routines, we often find change difficult. As an emotional eater you have probably come to use food as a habit to cope with a variety of situations. Please do not beat yourself up about this. Once upon a time the use of food to cope with emotions was probably helpful, for example, when you were a child and had less under-standing than you do now, or as an adult, you got short term comfort from food for a while and then it turned into an, almost unconscious, coping mechanism for everything.

The problem with routines and habits is that you might be hiding much of your beautiful and precious self. For example you might say, 'I always wear those jeans when I go out,' or 'I am always available to listen,' but these kinds of tight and rigid definitions can keep us from shining more of our light into the world. The good news is that we are all fully capable of change.

✍ Journal about some of your habits, routines and common rigid thoughts. Ask yourself if you would be willing to change any of these.

The first step is to get comfortable with change. In the first instance we are not going to look at food or emotional eating at all. We can start by thinking about making small changes in any area of our lives, so that we can begin to feel safe with change. Often we fear change because it is different from our usual way of being. We need to learn that change is safe.

The challenge: Do Something Different Today and every day for the next week. For example:

- If you usually wear your watch on your right wrist, switch it to the left.
- Take a different route when you walk or drive.
- If you usually listen to the radio when you eat breakfast, turn it off.
- If you take sugar in your tea, try it without.
- If you stand up when eating your breakfast start to sit down at the table.
- If you usually listen to the same CD over and over then change it and listen to something different.
- Wear odd socks under your jeans.

✎ Think of more changes. Then make the choice to actually do some of these changes. Notice how you feel about this change. Write about it in your journal. Can you see how the voice of fear turns up and tells you not to make the change? Even a really small change can feel like a massive challenge.

If you find playing with change difficult keep on giving yourself positive affirmations such as:

'It is safe to change;'
'I make changes easily;'
'Even though I am afraid I deeply and completely love and accept myself;'
'I am willing to change.'

This is about becoming more comfortable with change. Later we will be exploring alternative strategies to using food.

Rambunctious resources for change

♥ Cheri Huber. *Making a change for good. A guide to compassionate self-discipline.*

♥ Debbie Ford. *The 21 Day Consciousness Cleanse. A breakthrough program for connecting with your soul's deepest purpose.*

♥ Susan Jeffers. *Feel the fear and do it anyway.*

Chapter 9

Feelings and emotions

It is so common to talk about 'mind, body, and spirit' as a holistic path toward healing and change but often feelings and emotions get left out or are briefly glossed over.

Often for people who emotionally overeat, or comfort eat, it is a response to an unacknowledged feeling. Very often we 'think' rather than 'feel.' Our thoughts might be running riot and if we don't stop to feel our feelings it is likely that we'll turn to food because that is what we have always done. Very often we are afraid to 'feel.' Somewhere in our past we may have been taught that certain emotions were dangerous. Perhaps anger was not allowed or feeling happy meant that someone else would react with jealousy. As a child we may have repressed our emotions and turned to food as a way of coping, or stuffing them down.

We need to learn to allow our emotions to surface and to learn to sit with them and feel them

in the body without immediately heading to the refrigerator. Whilst writing this book I noticed that every so often I would find myself in the kitchen, looking in the cupboards as though something was going to jump out and save me. This was happening because I wasn't sitting down and allowing myself to feel what was going on. Instead I was getting stressed and overwhelmed with the writing process, trying to look after the house, walking the dog and being a 'good wife.' Instead of pausing to feel the emotion and sense it in my body, I was trying to escape. Knowing that this can happen is a lifeline because I was able STOP and remind myself to just 'be' with my Self and my feelings for a while. When I felt anxious or overwhelmed I chose to go for a walk, or weed my garden for 15 minutes, or sit and taste a cup of herbal tea.

It is safe to feel. All emotions are safe and acceptable.
The first step is to get comfortable with recognizing and naming our emotions/feelings. This may sound strange but many of us don't have a feelings vocabulary, especially when it comes to emotions that we have labeled as 'bad.'

Here are a few emotions:

Anger
Guilt
Dismay
Happiness
Safety
Hopelessness
Boredom
Irritation
Joy
Security
Panic
Worthlessness
Frustration
Love
Comfort
Anxiety
Sorrow
Jealousy
Excitement
Peace
Shame
Overwhelm
Impatience
Serenity
Compassion

Stopping to feel an emotion does not mean you have to act out from that emotion. In fact, being conscious of an emotion means we can consciously decide how to act from it. For example, anger doesn't need to result in violence or verbal abuse. Once you allow yourself to feel you can choose how to react. As with watching your thoughts you will come to realize that you are not your emotions. Feeling anger does not make you 'bad' and feeling compassion does not make you 'good.' As an observer of your thoughts and feelings you become empowered. Suppressing or denying the emotions is common practice in the modern world. Many of us fear our emotions or fear what might happen if we allow them to surface.

Investigate your feelings

Have a look at the list of feelings above. Set aside 10 to 15 minutes in a quiet place where you feel safe and won't be distracted. Read one of the words and then close your eyes. If thoughts begin to flood in bring yourself back to your breath, watch the thoughts as an impartial observer and let them go. Repeat the word to yourself. Next scan your body with your awareness, from your feet upwards; notice any places where you feel 'blocked' or irritated. It is important to understand that emotions are linked to physical sensations in the body. Taking time to see how emotions and physical sensations are linked can help us to become more aware in life and less likely to just head for food when we 'feel something.'

For example, when experiencing worry and despair the following comes up for me:

Worry – tightness in my chest, shallow breathing in my lungs, shoulders moving up toward my ears and curling forwards as if to protect my heart. Nervous feeling in my stomach, like whirlpools or unpleasant energy. Memories of abusive situations. Feeling of wanting to run away and hide.

Despair – remembering times of hopelessness and anguish, aloneness and sorrow. Breathing becoming fast and intense. Knots of tension in my chest/heart. Feeling as if I want to go and comfort myself with food to fill the emptiness inside.

When experiencing gratitude and joy the following comes up for me:

Gratitude – openness in my heart, deep and slow belly breaths, relaxed shoulders which are down and back so that my chest opens. Feeling an interconnection with people and things in my life that I am grateful for. A sense of oneness and harmony. A positive energy, a feeling of vitality vibrating in my body. A powerful sense of love for all that I am and all that I have.

Joy – energetic happiness, open heart, deep breathing that seems to fill my whole body. A sense of openness of mind, a letting go of any worry, a deep freedom to simply 'be' joy. My body feels really vibrant and expansive and tingling with waves of energy. The feeling that 'anything is possible' comes over me.

✎ Take time to write about your experience with sitting and feeling an emotion. Use color, describe sensations, write about the stream of thoughts that might come. Investigate as deeply as feels comfortable.

Emotions, all emotions whether comfortable/uncomfortable, positive/negative, can help us to connect, to be empathic and compassionate with ourselves and with other people. We begin to realize that we 'have' emotions but that we are not our emotions; they simply arise within the vast awareness. Being aware of emotions, being witness to them prevents us from suppressing and denying them – instead we allow them to come up and notice that they are just another thought form that can be let go of. In this way we realize that we do not have to be the victims of emotion, we can choose how to respond to an emotion rather than acting on it unconsciously. We realize that when we are aware of emotions we have a choice over how we respond – in this way we can become more centered and less fearful, more confident to be able to deal with life experiences in a calm and detached manner.

Instead of being caught up, overwhelmed, governed and pushed about by our emotions, through inner exploration we can learn to observe and be aware of our emotions and then to understand their nature. In this way we can learn to manage our lives more calmly – by becoming more aware of our emotions and understanding how best to respond to them. We begin to learn that we don't have to cope by using food; we can choose other, more loving, ways of being.

A good way to learn to deal immediately with powerful emotions such as rage or burning desire is to close your eyes and imagine being soothed by a gentle breeze or cooling rain and imagine inner turmoil being blown or washed away. It can also be helpful to write about your emotions in your journal in order to let them out and let them go. Feelings can also seem to carry energy, you might find that going for a walk or dancing around to your favorite music after doing feelings work can help move this energy around and release it.

Many people have said that our emotions are really all just aspects of love and fear. Letting go of fear and embracing love, of others and ourselves can lead to a sense of freedom.

'Fear contracts the heart. Its worries and anxieties stop the flow of love. Do we really want to live in fear?'
~ Jack Kornfield

Love of ourselves leads to love of others. The Buddha said, 'Like a caring mother holding and guarding the life of her only child, so with a boundless heart of lovingkindness, hold yourself and all beings as your beloved children.'

It is often said that love and fear cannot coexist. Where one is, the other cannot also be, e.g. if you are in a situation where you are filled with immense joy and then suddenly you are overtaken by fear, the joy (love) is gone but this also works the other way, if we are in fear we can turn to the love within. We can learn to make an active choice to be in love and not fear in every situation we encounter. In this way we can find inner peace, if we could all do this then perhaps world peace really could be inevitable!

If you have a thought or feeling that you have decided in the past to label as 'bad' or 'unacceptable,' such as anger or jealousy, then you may well turn to negative self-talk or eating as a way to punish yourself. The aim is to catch the thought about anger or jealousy and realize it is just a thought, it isn't 'bad' and it doesn't make us bad to have those thoughts. Then we see there is no need to stuff down those feelings with food. We also don't have to cover those feelings up with 'I feel fat' – we can, instead, silently acknowledge, or write in our journals: 'I feel angry about x, y, z,' or 'I feel jealous.' This releases us from the need to stuff down the thought and judge it as bad. We can also look inside and see if we have a need. Do we need to acknowledge ourselves for our achievements, find a safe friend to talk to, take a rest, etc?

✎ What feelings do you find most difficult? Which emotions have you labeled as 'bad,' can you begin to release that label and see that an emotion is neither good nor bad?

Check in with your 'hunger;' what are you hungry for? It might well be food but it may also be a 'need.' It takes fearless courage to sit with a feeling and ask ourselves what we need rather than just jumping for food. Often it feels unbearable to sit with feelings; it can seem that we might explode. Loving ourselves is crucial at this time. Sitting with anger, anxiety, jealousy, joy, overwhelm, even for just 30 seconds, can lead us to deep realizations if we let them. Feelings can be a flashlight for us. They can shine a light on past things that we may have squashed down, it can be painful to bring these things up – but it's not a case of dwelling on them, simply freeing ourselves from the past so that the now can be peaceful and not constantly a place of using food to hide.

Stress and overwhelm were huge triggers for my overeating. I was a nervous child; I wanted to make everything ok for everyone. I wanted to do what I could to help at home. My dad used to travel a lot for business and I was aware of my mum's sadness and her overwhelm too. I tried to be good and helpful but I was often anxious and felt responsible for everything that happened and any accident. I remember I used to say 'sorry' a lot, for everything even things like spilling my drink. Throughout school I had the same feelings and then I went on to be self-employed at a very young age. I had to be all departments: accounts, marketing, advertising, copywriting, etc. The people pleasing and the anxiety were a common factor. I really was doing my best to just 'be everything' and never ask for help or support. Looking back it hurts, I needed to love myself, to care for myself, to be able to ask for help and support and genuine friendship.

I always also had a deep love for the Divine, as I began to meditate more and be mindful of my feelings, I began to see a larger picture; I began to realize my worth. When feelings are squashed with food, life becomes very narrow, we miss a lot, and we live from the black/white rather than the full rainbow. Through sitting with my anxiety I realized that I could always be there for myself. That I will never leave myself. This drew me deep into meditating on 'who am I?' Who is this 'I' who never leaves, who always cares, who always loves me, who is love?

In *When women stop hating their bodies,* Jane Hirschmann and Carol Munter write about the urge to eat when we are not hungry, which is generally triggered by one of three situations 1. When we feel in danger of being overwhelmed by our feelings 2. When we feel the guilt that follows 'forbidden' feelings or thoughts and 3. When we feel like a failure in any context.' If we know this we can begin to stop, breathe and respond to ourselves with self-care and not food.

🖋 Investigate some of your own 'hungers' and the need that might be behind them.

Even now, Mondays are my challenging day with food. Chris, my husband, leaves in the morning after we've had a fun weekend together and I feel: Lost, Bored, Lonely, Alone, Overwhelmed that I have to work, Stubborn. Basically I feel a lot of things but my brain thinks – just eat, eat the feelings away. It happens most Monday mornings but after living with Chris now for over two years I know the score and so I have a toolkit of things to help me. It can be horrible to have to sit and observe those feelings, it feels like death sometimes but after practice I can do it. I often go and walk Freddy-dog and then I come home in a calm and conscious mindset and can begin work. The feelings often shift and change very quickly, allowing peace to filter through. Keep practicing, keep noticing, and keep making conscious shifts.

Emotions often point towards needs or desires

While you were doing the emotions work you may have noticed that certain emotions were linked to an inner need. Often when we are not allowing our feelings and emotions to speak to us we don't listen to what they are asking. We know there is a 'need' deep down there somewhere but because we don't sit and feel our feelings we kid ourselves into believing that the need is food (and sometimes, if we are actually hungry the need is food!).

Once you are comfortable with sitting and feeling your feelings and emotions you can begin to ask yourself 'what do I really need?' Don't try to force the answers, let them arise and be open to hearing them. If you feel sad you might need a hug. If you feel angry you might need to talk to someone about it or move the energy by going for a walk or vacuuming the house.

Sometimes emotional eating is triggered by feelings we might think of as positive such as happiness. If you feel happy it might be that you need to shout about it and share it with the world. This might feel difficult since culturally we are not generally taught that celebrating our happiness and joy is acceptable. This is changing, thankfully. We need to share our joy. For me personally in my past, I would eat to prevent myself from feeling happy, because being happy around certain people in my past life wasn't safe; they got jealous and then usually ignored me or got angry. Now I have safe friends and we love to share in each other's joy. We encourage one another to share positive experiences and joy. You do not need to hide your happiness, or cover it up with eating; it is safe to be filled with joy. You can choose to talk to people who will be happy with you, or do a private happy dance to allow the happy energy to flow, or post your joy on a forum or blog.

Sometimes it might seem that no one is there to fulfill your need. This is when it is so important to learn that you can fulfill your needs by learning to love on yourself. You are a precious and empowered being and you can look within. This isn't selfish, this is vital.

This poem, *The Guesthouse*, teaches us that all feelings are valid and all feelings can be teachers that need to be welcomed and listened to:

The Guesthouse

This being human is a guest house.
Every morning a new arrival.

A joy, a depression, a meanness,
some momentary awareness comes
as an unexpected visitor.

Welcome and entertain them all!
Even if they're a crowd of sorrows,
who violently sweep your house
empty of its furniture,
still, treat each guest honorably.
He may be clearing you out
for some new delight.

The dark thought, the shame, the malice,
meet them at the door laughing,
and invite them in.
Be grateful for whoever comes,
because each has been sent
as a guide from beyond.

~ Rumi
(*The Essential Rumi*, versions by Coleman Barks)

As a child I was told, 'I want, gets nothing.' I internalized this as meaning it was not ok to have needs and desires. It took lots of inner work in order to believe that I was allowed to have wants, needs, and desires. I also began to understand that I could give myself what I wanted a lot of the time. I didn't have to wait to be bought flowers or to give myself permission to rest, change bank accounts, look at new jobs etc. Be empowered, allow yourself to have needs, allow yourself to fulfill your needs. Be gentle with yourself as you practice.

🖉 How do you feel about having needs?

Rambunctious resources for the exploration of feelings and emotions

- ♥ Cheri Huber. *There is nothing wrong with you. Going beyond self-hate. A compassionate process for learning to accept yourself exactly as you are.*
- ♥ Debbie Ford. *The dark side of the light chasers. Reclaiming your power, creativity, brilliance and dreams.*
- ♥ Tara Brach. *Radical Acceptance. Embracing your life with the heart of a Buddha.*
- ♥ Shakti Gawain. *The Path Of Transformation. How healing ourselves can change the world.*
- ♥ Caroline Myss. *Why people don't heal and how they can.*
- ♥ Mark Williams, John Teasdale, Zindel Segal and Jon Kabat-Zinn. *The mindful way through depression. Freeing yourself from chronic unhappiness.*

Chapter 10

Investigate your food beliefs

Old food beliefs need to be challenged in order for change to be possible. It may take months to challenge what you were taught as a child but old food beliefs need to be investigated and busted open with compassion.

Here are a few common things you may have heard as a child:

'You are such a good girl for eating everything on your plate;'

'If you don't eat everything on that plate you won't get any ice-cream;'

'It is bad to waste food, there are starving children in the world;'

'If you are a good girl Mummy will buy you some chocolate;'

'Don't be sad, don't cry, here are some sweets to make you feel better;'

'Take that angry look off your face or you won't be getting any pudding.'

Food may never have just been food in your household. It may have been a bribe, a reward, used as punishment. You learned that even if you were full you had to finish what was on your plate, so you learned not to listen to the wisdom of your body. Your body was wrong, the plate was right. You developed emotional eating and comfort eating habits and now it seems such a challenge to break out of those habits, but it can be done!

✐ Write about what food meant in your household. Investigate some of the beliefs you may have internalized. Do you still hold these beliefs?

This morning I watched Freddy-dog eat about half of his breakfast and then walk away. He didn't want any more, he frequently does this and will go back to it later when he's hungry. He's a great teacher. Food is there to fuel him, I doubt he has any complex food beliefs!

Food myths and beliefs we were taught can be questioned and changed now. It can take time and patience but change is possible. We can begin to tune back in to the wisdom of the body, to allow feelings, to change our habit of rewarding, and punishing, ourselves with food.

🖉 Take your journal and question these beliefs, are they true? Is it YOUR belief or someone else's? Can you think of new beliefs and ways to break the habit?

You are not 'good' or 'bad' for eating everything on your plate. Eating has nothing to do with your innate goodness. Tune into that. Experiment with mindful eating (which we will be looking at in the next section) so that you can start tasting and feeling food in your body, learning to listen for signals that you have had enough. Just investigate these thoughts and beliefs.

When I was doing my eating disorders training course we were set an assignment to go out and buy some food and then to throw it away. The uproar in the classroom was immense. We were asked to discuss our reaction and question it. I had a couple of things going on – I wasn't earning great money so that was an issue, until the tutor reminded me I could probably pick something up for 20p (I grumbled and then dug into my purse to see how many 1p and 2p coins I had hiding). There was the deeper reaction to wasting food too. I had been taught that was bad and so if I did it I was obviously bad too! Ha ha. A myth. I also asked the tutor, 'If there is a homeless person sitting next to the bin can I give them the food?' I was told 'no,' SIGH. My grandparents had been through a pretty tough time in prison camps during the war and food was highly prized. All of this was coming up because I was going to spend 20p on a sweet and throw it away. Some people in the class just couldn't bring themselves to do it. Understandable, but interesting. I did it and it pushed me to go on and question a whole lot more.

We finish food when we are not hungry because it would be a waste to throw it out. Is it true that it would be a waste to throw it out? Are we human dustbins? If we eat the food when we are not hungry then our bodies probably don't need it, so what happens? We probably get bloated and uncomfortable and then this brings up more difficult feelings. If the food on our plate cannot be wrapped up and stored in the refrigerator until tomorrow and we don't want to eat it now then throwing it away is a kind thing to do and not wasteful at all.

🖉 Just take time to notice your beliefs. Write about them. Question them. Make changes, little ones. Love yourself while you do this.

When I wrote a blog post about this topic, I got many comments on my Facebook page. It is an emotive subject, particularly food-waste. There is no question that far too much food is wasted in the Western world. However, an individual who is struggling with emotional eating, especially in the early stages, needs to be able to let go of the guilt that can be associated with not finishing what they may have begun eating. Guilt is a major problem for a lot of women who eat emotionally and it is incredibly destructive and can prevent healing. The early phases of exploring emotional eating are very tender and old habits and beliefs can keep us stuck. Over time, when emotional eating is not such a problem, we begin to learn and listen to what we wish to eat and how much, and food waste becomes less of an issue.

Issues with food and eating represent a serious opportunity to delve into the depth of who you are. Diving into these deep feelings, although intensely challenging, brings about a vast freedom and opens up waves of sweetness if you are prepared to be fearlessly honest with yourself.

✐ Who would I be without my emotional eating?

Here is an excerpt from one of my own journals, from my early 20s:

What would it be like to just let go? To relax? To trust? What would that be like? I don't fear the tsunami of emotions and feelings, or perhaps I do? I fear just eating and not living my life. I fear hiding myself away forever and missing the beauty. Who would I be if I just let go of this tendency to compulsively eat when I feel overwhelmed? Would I fall into the arms of my True Nature that which always is, yet never seems to be? Perhaps eating actually attempts to keep me from that which I AM. Perhaps if I stop to feel the overwhelm, I'll get past it and then I'll realize I'm breathtakingly me and that I am awesome. Perhaps I really do fear shining my light out into the world, just like Marianne Williamson wrote:

'Our deepest fear is not that we are inadequate. Our deepest fear is that we are powerful beyond measure. It is our light, not our darkness, that most frightens us. We ask ourselves, who am I to be brilliant, gorgeous, talented, fabulous? Actually, who are you not to be? You are a child of God. Your playing small doesn't serve the world. There's nothing enlightened about shrinking so that other people won't feel insecure around you. You were born to manifest the glory of God that is within you. It is not just in some of us; it is in everyone. And as we let our own light shine, we unconsciously give other people permission to do the same. As we're liberated from our own fear, our presence automatically

liberates others.'
~ Marianne Williamson, *A Return To Love* 1993

This was a turning point for me, the realization that there was a conflict between being free from emotional eating and staying an emotional eater. When you look at this conflict it can, initially, seem strange. You might say, 'Of course I want to be free.' Sit more deeply with that. Ask yourself, 'who would I be if I stopped comfort eating?'

✐ Grab your journal and be fearlessly honest with yourself. List the pros and cons of letting go and allowing healing from your comfort eating. Do this gently with no self judgment.

Here are a few ideas, delve into yourself for your own limiting beliefs.

Pros / Gains of freeing myself from emotional eating:

If I were to be free from emotional eating it might mean...

- I'll have more space in my mind, I won't just be thinking about being dependent on food;
- Freedom from shame and guilt;
- My friendships and relationships will be better;
- My self-esteem will be higher;
- My world will be brighter;
- I'll have more confidence to look at other fears and hurdles in my life;
- Freedom to live my best life;
- I'll have more time to do the things I really love.

Cons / Sacrifices of freeing myself from emotional eating:

If I were to be free from emotional eating it might mean...

- I might feel deprived of certain foods;
- I might have to actually deal with problems in my relationship;
- I will have to face difficult feelings around a childhood trauma;
- I will have to be more assertive and less of a people pleaser;
- That there is nothing blocking me from my dreams and that is frightening;
- I'll have more time and I don't know how I will fill it, what if I suddenly realize I am totally alone?

We need to look at what might be keeping us stuck in emotional eating. This is very empowering because then we can look at the fears and how we use food to sabotage ourselves from living a full life. With this knowledge you can expand and go beyond the blocks, you might want to see a counselor or therapist, or speak with a coach to help you get past these self-limiting beliefs. Or you may be able to journal and question your way through them with quiet time and introspection. Remember to observe the thoughts, they are just thoughts, they can be changed, they are not who you are. Remember to write your insights down, this gets them out of your head!

You were not born to simply be on a continuous diet cycle. You were born to live your life in your particular, beautiful, way. When obsession with food dies down, space opens up for investigation with creativity; you might want to look at new jobs, re-training, relationships, and travel. This can be frightening, but you won't choose to go back to food because the urge will be too strong, once you have opened the doorway to the soul and caught a glimpse of Spirit it is impossible to forget what you have seen.

🖋 It really is time to open yourself up. You can see how your emotional eating might be holding you back. Ask yourself, if you were not worrying about your emotional eating, what would you most like to do? Don't let the mind get too involved. Close your eyes, breathe and drop down into your heart area and feel your body. Write a list of all the things you would love to do. For example:

- ♥ Go out to lunch with my friend;
- ♥ Try out that salsa dancing class that keeps being advertised;
- ♥ Go and study for that course I have always wanted to do;
- ♥ Begin going to the creative writing workshop that happens in the local library;
- ♥ Buy some new clothes;
- ♥ Go bungee jumping;
- ♥ Join a painting class;
- ♥ Go to a support group;
- ♥ Start going to yoga;
- ♥ Eat dinner at the table with my family;
- ♥ Take a holiday;
- ♥ Learn a new language;
- ♥ Spend more time in nature;
- ♥ Share more joy and smile more!

Gently explore your dreams and desires. Look at your list. Pick something from that list that feels the safest for you and allow yourself the pleasure of doing it. If you need support then could you ask a friend to join you? I had wanted to go to yoga classes for years but I just couldn't get myself there, I was afraid, it was new, I didn't know anyone there. I decided to email the teacher in advance, I was vulnerable, and I said I was nervous – she replied and I felt so at ease. The class was so peaceful and there was a lot of emphasis on being with the breath and mindfulness, which, as we have seen, is really helpful for many life situations. If I had let the fear win I would not have experienced the profound pleasure of yoga. It is easy to hold ourselves back and stay with what is familiar but it can be tiring to live a life that is full of anxiety and so focused on keeping you in a narrow definition of who you are. Remember, you are not your emotional eating patterns – you are so much more than just that. Allow yourself to slowly expand into new experiences. Some you might love and others you won't like as much but you will never know if you don't take that step. Do it lovingly and gently. Let your soul sing.

Conflict around shape change

Another conflict that comes up for many women is body shape. Your shape may, or may not change when you stop emotionally eating. How do you feel about that? After doing the pros and cons exercise above we can move on and do shape conflict work.

✎ Take your journal and list all the positive and negative qualities that come to mind when thinking about a woman who is slim and one who is larger. This is not an exercise of judgment, so please keep your heart open when you look at what comes up for you. This is an exercise at looking deep into our own conditioned beliefs. It can help us to uncover some of the thinking patterns that might be unconsciously keeping us stuck and blocking our healing. Here are a few things that often come up:

Slim is:
Positives: attractive, popular, in control, confident, intelligent, lucky, pretty, healthy, assertive;
Negatives: controlling, cold, nasty, not-understanding, self-centered, threatening, only likes other thin people, selfish and not giving, bad listener.
Larger is:
Positives: nurturing, sensitive, compassionate, easy going,

easy to talk to, fun, giving, good listener;
Negatives: lazy, no self control, no willpower, unhealthy, no self respect, not bright.

🖉 Is this list true? Do you know people who don't fit that mould? Can you see how your own judgments might be keeping you small? Do you worry that if you change shape to get smaller or larger then people might think these things of you?

It is our duty to break the chain of these kinds of thoughts. Often our ancestry has programmed these thoughts and judgments, they are our family beliefs and not really ours. It is time to fearlessly look at our beliefs and decide to change them, to become more caring, compassionate and accepting. I know some incredibly fit, healthy, vivacious people who are larger than a size 14. I also know some slimmer people who are unhealthy and unkind. I also know beautifully sweet and kind and healthy slim people and unhealthy, unkind larger people – BUT we are all humans, we all have feelings, we struggle, we feel pain and we deserve compassion and a non-judgmental attitude. It starts with how we judge ourselves. It comes back to learning how to love ourselves – this helps our judgments to dissipate and we find that we become more compassionate to others as well as ourselves.

Recently I had an email from a lovely lady. She wrote:

One thing I do know that I have to overcome – whenever I lose weight, I get to a certain point and start thinking I'm not worthy to be thin so I start putting it back on. I also have something my mom said for years, 'Thin people look their age faster than fat people and you don't want to be too thin in case you get sick.'

This is a portion of my response:

I wanted to respond to your note about weight loss and feeling worthy, this is really common and really important to address. It is great that you already have insight and can hear some of your mom's past conditioning about being thin, knowing this is powerful because it gives you something to work with. I suggest writing down all the positives and negatives that you might feel about healing your emotional heating (or weight loss). It is amazing how many deep-rooted beliefs we might have. It is important to do this work compassionately and gently but also with fierce honesty. When I had problems with binge eating it was because I was a people pleaser and found it so hard to say 'no' so I stuffed myself instead. I realized that in order to change I had to learn to be assertive and that was hard...but I took it in small steps. I also used to eat (and still sometimes do) when I felt overwhelmed and anxious – it was a way of zoning out, so I had to learn to be able to sit with the discomfort of anxiety rather than run to the food.

With regards to weight loss and then not feeling worthy – this is where extreme self-compassion is needed! I would suggest you spend some time each day doing something you love, just for you. Watch whether feelings of guilt come up and then keep affirming that you are worthy of feeling happy and worthy of pleasure. If we are conscious of these patterns we can break the chain of past conditioning, not just for ourselves but for future generations. We are all worthy of joy and being the best we can be...but it can be so hard! I know I still struggle with worth and feeling guilty but I make a conscious effort to change the self-talk in my mind. I try to treat myself the way I would treat my best friend, or a precious child. It just takes a bit of continued practice. Please be gentle with yourself whilst you explore these thoughts, feelings and beliefs.

Whilst doing this work you might feel as though there are

three separate people in the equation:

The real YOU, the non-judgmental, peaceful observer;
The part of you that wants to be free of emotional eating;
The part of you that wants to hang on to the emotional eating.

It is really important to take time to do this conflict work because it gives you the chance to see what might be blocking your healing. Something powerful that works for a lot of people is to imagine the two parts that are in conflict. Have a dialogue with each part. You might want to draw or write about the feelings, thoughts, emotions, colors and anything else that comes up. Be non-judgmental as you do this. Be the loving observer that you are. What does each part look like? How old is that part? Ask each part what their needs are, what their goals are, what their hurts are. Reassure them that they are both loved and respected. Even the part that doesn't want to let go of the emotional eating will have valid reasons – this part is often young and may just need to be validated, loved and respected by you. Don't squash her down. The needs of the part that wants to emotionally eat can be honored and you can fulfill those needs without food once you know what they are. It could be that you need to learn to be assertive and say 'no' to things, or perhaps take more breaks, walks, meditate. She'll tell you what she needs and at the core it will be love. You can begin to learn how to love yourself without the food.

Once you have dialogued with the two parts of you that are in conflict you can imagine them coming together, let them embrace. Bring them into your heart.

✎ Journal about this experience. It is important that you know that it is safe to stop emotionally eating and safe to use self-love as a tool for healing. This process can take time and if you are finding it particularly difficult you may also want to enlist the help of a therapist. Be compassionate as you delve into these feelings.

Challenging thoughts like this can work on many levels. For instance, I had to work really hard on my own belief that I was not worthy of feeling happiness. If I felt happy I would feel guilty and so I would start to eat rather than show my happiness to the world. Of course the eating only gave me a moment of happiness, which was followed by guilt and sorrow. In some ways I got stuck in that because sorrow, sadness, struggle, suffering and depression were safe. It wasn't until I was studying for a counseling certificate in psychosynthesis and I had to have personal psychotherapy as part of the course, that I realized I had to break the chain, the ancestral chain, the chains of old family beliefs that were no longer serving anyone.

Suffering is something I remember hearing my grandparents talk a lot about. As I grew up I internalized various messages about suffering. In addition to this, I grew up knowing about the terror that my grandparents went through in World War Two. Both sets of my grandparents had lived in Poland. They were all in various camps during the war. One of my grandmothers was sent in a cattle truck to Siberia to a camp with horrible conditions. As a child, this was difficult to hear about and know about, although it was important as it represented part of my story and my heritage. As I discovered in my psychotherapy sessions, I was experiencing a form of survivor's guilt. Deep down, I honestly believed that I was not worthy of feeling happiness because of all the pain my grandparents went through. The underlying message in my head that played on a loop was 'who am I to be happy?'

In one of my sessions, my therapist, Heather, asked me to draw a picture of myself and it was then that I realized I had to 'break the chains.' The image that I drew of myself was really shadowy and dark and I was dragging heavy black chains around with me, they extended backwards and deep, deep into the soil. They represented years of ancestral suffering and hardship. At the top of my drawing I colored a curious bright light, and as I talked through my therapy I realized that the light was the light of hope and awareness. Deep within me I knew that I could, if I chose to, break the chains, break the suffering and decide that I was worthy of happiness and decide to share my joy more in the world, fearlessly, courageously and without reservation.

That was just the beginning. It took time for me to experiment with joy. Friends left my life because they didn't like the new, happier, more assertive me, the 'me' who cared about myself as well as others. Still now I sometimes struggle and head for food when I feel joy – because I think all of us, in a way carry some kind of feeling about being 'too happy' when there is so much suffering in the world. I have come to learn to keep on questioning the voice that says, 'who am I to be happy?,' 'who am I not to be?' I reply. Does my suffering serve the world? If I am happy it does not mean that I do not also hold compassion and sorrow in my heart for the sorrow in the world. I see both. I see the whole and I truly believe that until we can share our joys the world will not heal from its suffering. We have to be the loving examples. We have to break the chain.

You might be thinking, 'it is too hard!' Well, Rome wasn't built in a day, but small steps lead to big differences. As it says in the *Tao Teh Ching*, 'the journey of a thousand miles begins with a single step.' If we, each of us, took our small steps then we could cause a revolution. It IS worth the effort and if we do it together we can support one another along the way.

This is an affirmation that I use when I need a boost, often I'll journal my affirmations but I'll also use them spoken out loud:

I deeply and completely love and accept myself NOW, as I am today. I choose to be compassionate with myself. I am gentle and supportive with myself as I take the journey toward change. It is safe for me to be happy, it is safe for me to shine and take care of myself. I take time to listen to my body and my True Self and I choose to fulfill my authentic needs.

Life does not suddenly become paradise when you are thin or hell when you are large. Our feelings, thoughts and criticism send us to the hell place and self-love is the angel that can bring us back to the heaven of the present, delicious moment. No matter what size or shape you are it is crucial to practice radical self-love and nurturing. You are worthy and when you care about your worth you become more loving and in touch with the worth of those around you and you begin to see how badly people treat themselves. We can be part of the change. Women regularly bond by talking about weight and diets – let's change that, let's become women who can go deep together and look at the true feelings and needs beneath the supposed need to become thin.

Food and sex

When women begin to look at patterns, feelings and needs they often find that their eating and feelings of sexuality, sexual power and sexual beauty are all linked. Many, but not all women who suffer with emotional eating have been through some kind of sexual trauma in their lives. Many women have certainly had incidences of being 'sexualized' or seen as sexy by men in a way that they found to be uncomfortable. Also, many women have been brought up to believe that being sexy was, in some way, a bad thing or dangerous.

Food can be used to suppress feelings of sexiness. Unconsciously, we might be eating to weigh ourselves down with protective layers, squash our sexuality, keep us somehow invisible as women, or we might eat to become bigger and more powerful, more able to exist in a place where men might be dominant and femininity is seen a weak. Sometimes, we eat in order to make ourselves less attractive. At other times, we might feel that our battle with food is lessening and we begin to feel sexy and great, regardless of our body size/shape -then feelings of guilt or shame come up, are we supposed to feel sexy? And then we sabotage our good feelings with food.

It is a complicated web when it comes to food and sex. Some women turn to food because they have been taught that it is not ok to be sexy or have sexual feelings or to enjoy their own, beautiful bodies. There are still so many taboos when it comes to sex. Thankfully these are lifting slowly, but ancestral beliefs are something we seem to carry deep within us. It is these beliefs that we must challenge for ourselves and change for future generations.

I was brought up in a Catholic household. My parents didn't teach me anything about sex. My Catholic, all girls, school taught me almost nothing – just the bare minimum needed to pass my biology GCSE. Nothing about feelings around sexuality, nothing about the beauty of the female body, the sacredness of the Divine Goddess within. Sex before marriage and having sex with more than one partner were just not acceptable in my family lineage. Can you imagine my confusion, shame and guilt? I had to sift through so many beliefs that were not my beliefs. My Soul had to find her own peace. I traversed a rocky road on my journey toward embracing myself as a wonderful, sexual being. I made painful mistakes along the way. I ate, and sometimes starved, my guilt and shame and also my pleasure and feelings of 'badness' around sexuality. Even now I am still investigating my sexual nature.

These feelings of sexuality can infuse into us in many ways. Often we do not dress the way that we wish to, for fear of looking too sexy or passionate, or we dress to enhance our femininity and have feelings to shame come up which need to be loved and investigated and let go of.

The whole issue is a large one. You might want to investigate this with a therapist or take as much time as you need with your journal. This is a vast subject area, read about the idea of female Goddess, of Divinity, and read about Tantra. Look into your belief systems, are those your beliefs or just learned beliefs. Be fearlessly honest with yourself. Question what you were taught, re-write your own story. Love yourself through this process of exploration. We are sexual beings and that is ok. Work to discover your own flavor of sexuality and grow toward owning that.

✐ Take time to investigate your own feelings toward sex and sexuality. Can you re-write some of your old rules and stories?

Rambunctious resources for the exploration of sexiness

- ♥ Lisa Clark. *Sassy. The Go-For-It Girl's Guide to becoming mistress of your destiny.*
- ♥ Valerie Brooks. *Tantric Awakening. A woman's initiation into the path of ecstasy.*
- ♥ Regena Thomashauer. *Mama Gena's School of Womanly Arts. Using the power of pleasure to have your way with the world.*

Chapter 11

Mindful eating

How often, when you are eating, are you truly aware of what is on the plate or how the food tastes? Do you eat whilst watching the TV, or listening to the radio, or do you read the newspaper whilst you chow-down? 'Mindful eating' describes a nonjudgmental awareness of physical and emotional sensations associated with eating.

Here is an experiment for you: Next time you are having a meal, sit down at a table that you have specially laid. Before you begin eating look at the plate in front of you, notice what is on it. Don't be judgmental or critical; just notice what is there. Then notice how you feel in your body physically, is there any tightness, lightness, physical feelings? Then notice how you feel emotionally – are you anxious, anticipating, sad, stressed from a hard day? Just notice it all. Then put some food into your mouth, put your knife and fork down and chew the food at least ten times. Notice how it feels and tastes, notice your thoughts – which might be, 'this is such a stupid exercise,' just notice and do it anyway. Then continue to eat and notice all the time. See what happens. Do you find that you are full quicker than normal? Do you notice that actually you didn't really like what you were eating? Do you notice new flavors and textures?

🖊 After you finish eating take some time to journal about your experience.

Studies have shown that mindful eating is significantly associated with decreases in binge eating, depression and perceived stress. Feeling mindfully connected to the body and mind, being aware of physical feelings/sensations in the body and emotional states and feelings such as anger, sadness, joy, etc has been linked to healthier eating patterns, reduced food quantity, increased food quality, positive feelings toward the body and general wellbeing.

There is an American organization, 'The Center for Mindful Eating,' who have created the following Principles of Mindful Eating. http://www.tcme.org/principles.htm

Principles of Mindfulness:

- Mindfulness is deliberately paying attention, non-judgmentally.
- Mindfulness encompasses both internal processes and external environments.
- Mindfulness is being aware of what is present for you mentally, emotionally and physically in each moment.
- With practice, mindfulness cultivates the possibility of freeing yourself of reactive, habitual patterns of thinking, feeling and acting.
- Mindfulness promotes balance, choice, wisdom and acceptance of what is.

Mindful Eating is:

- Allowing yourself to become aware of the positive and nurturing opportunities that are available through food preparation and consumption by respecting your own inner wisdom.
- Choosing to eat food that is both pleasing to you and nourishing to your body by using all your senses to explore, savor and taste.
- Acknowledging responses to food (likes, neutral or dislikes) without judgment.
- Learning to be aware of physical hunger and satiety cues

to guide your decision to begin eating and to stop eating.

Someone Who Eats Mindfully:

- Acknowledges that there is no right or wrong way to eat but varying degrees of awareness surrounding the experience of food.
- Accepts that his/her eating experiences are unique.
- Is an individual who by choice, directs his/her awareness to all aspects of food and eating on a moment-by-moment basis.
- Is an individual who looks at the immediate choices and direct experiences associated with food and eating: not to the distant health outcome of that choice.
- Is aware of and reflects on the effects caused by unmindful eating.
- Experiences insight about how he/she can act to achieve specific health goals as he/she becomes more attuned to the direct experience of eating and feelings of health.
- Becomes aware of the interconnection of earth, living beings, and cultural practices and the impact of his/ her food choices has on those systems.

Mindfulness has also been successfully used to treat stress, anxiety, chronic pain and depression – all of which can contribute to emotional eating.

Please remember that mindfulness is loving, peaceful and non-judgmental! Mindfulness can also teach us about the inter-connection between beings and in life, it can help us to know that we are not alone.

For example: Sit down for ten minutes and really taste a cup of herbal tea. Feel the warmth of the mug in your hands and drink in the comfort of the hot liquid. Allow the moment to nurture you. The universe is in that mug of tea – the sun, rain, soil, plants, the farm workers and the shop assistants who sold it to you. The chain of life is mesmerizing. You may be taken on a long and powerful journey if you can really be mindful to that cup on tea.

Mindfulness can help to stop us from unconsciously eating. Eating mindfully brings you back to you, back to the moment and away from fearful thoughts or feelings and negative self-talk, it brings you back to the moment, back to the tastes, back to calm. Mindful eating does take practice, but don't give up. When I am stressed and don't remember to eat mindfully I often end up eating when really I just need a rest or a break or a walk. If I begin to eat mindfully I often stop mid-bite because I realize my true need is not the food at that moment.

At first as we become aware and mindful of our eating habits, the pain of the heightened awareness may make the problem seem 10000 times more painful. This is because we suddenly see what we are doing but are not quite ready to let go, the eating is not unconscious anymore – so a conflict or struggle can arise. This is why it is so important to be ultra gentle and non-judgmental with yourself as you explore mindful eating and mindfulness in general. Keep your thoughts on paper, often we do not realize how far we have come. Having a journal gives us useful reference points and we can use it to celebrate all the milestones on our personal journey.

Rambunctious resources for the exploration of mindful eating

- ♥ Thich Nhat Hanh. *Mindful eating, mindful life.*
- ♥ Susan Albers. *Eat, Drink, and be Mindful: How to End Your Struggle with Mindless Eating and Start Savoring Food with Intention and Joy.*
- ♥ Andrew Weiss. *Beginning mindfulness. Learning the way of awareness.*

♥ Mark Williams, John Teasdale, Zindel Segal and Jon Kabat-Zinn. *The mindful way through depression. Freeing yourself from chronic unhappiness.*

Chapter 12

Assertiveness skills and learning how to have healthy boundaries

Learning assertiveness skills is so important for those of us who over eat. If we don't have healthy boundaries, we are not loving ourselves. If we are not attending to our needs, our needs shout, we don't listen and we end up eating instead. It becomes a really painful cycle. Assertion is self-love, it is empowering. It is healing. However, it is also very challenging for many people. Like me, you may have been a people pleaser for years. You might be doing all that you can for others, for everyone other than yourself and it is likely that you are eating to fill the hole inside of yourself, in order to drown out your needs. You might be eating because you feel guilty for having needs! Learning how to be lovingly assertive is crucial, learning to lovingly say 'no' and not feel guilty about it is so fantastically liberating!

> Every time you say yes when you mean no, you are training yourself to deny your souls truth and to ignore your inner knowing.
> ~ Alice Bandy (in Debbie Ford's book, *The 21 day consciousness cleanse*)

How often have you said yes to something that you really didn't have the energy to do, or you really didn't feel good about doing? If you don't love yourself you are probably used to giving yourself away and saying yes to everyone but yourself. This may well leave you feeling exhausted and possibly resentful? It is SO important to learn to say no, to fill yourself up with love first and then decide on whether you can say yes to other requests for help/support. This isn't selfish. I used to be the queen of do, do, doing stuff for other people when really I just wanted some time for myself to be (after all we are human-beings not human-doings). I helped many other people's dreams come true and suddenly realized that my own dreams were hidden in the basement. I was 'too nice,' it didn't really dawn on me until I was forced to say no because I was too sick to get out of my bed! Please don't let it go that far!! Being NICE isn't always the most loving option. It can mean that Nothing Inside Cares Enough.

My very wise therapist, Heather, once said to me, 'Ani, a "no" can be as loving as a "yes".' I had equated NO with being 'bad' but as we learned earlier no just means no, it is the stories the mind and the inner critic tell us that make us believe it to be wrong.

Stop forcing yourself to do things you really don't want to do. Look into your heart, be honest with yourself and choose what is most nourishing for you in the moment. Honor your needs; it isn't selfish, it is necessary. You cannot help others if you are burnt out, exhausted and resentful. Fill yourself up with self-love and then you will have enough to give to others without feeling depleted.

Say to yourself: 'I make loving and nourishing choices for myself,' 'I lovingly take care of my own needs.'

For years you may not have had healthy boundaries, but it is never too late to start. You may be worried that friends and family might react badly to your newfound voice? If you can, talk to those closest to you and explain that you are taking some time for yourself. If they really love and respect you they will understand, even if they grumble a bit. Lovely Heather also taught me that I could say to people, 'I am not doing this against you, I am doing it for myself.' When I began having healthy boundaries, some of my friendships did dissolve and drift away and it was upsetting but ultimately I can see these were not healthy or authentic relationships. I still love those people in my heart and wish them well but I am glad that I made the choice to love myself enough to say 'no' to things I really didn't feel good about doing, or didn't have the energy to do. Having healthy boundaries helps us to create space in our heart and will often mean we turn less to food for comfort.

Bending the truth was something I used to do a lot because I could not say 'no' to people or requests. Instead of just saying 'no' I felt like I had to give a valid excuse. Then I would feel terrible for lying and I would go and eat because of the guilt, and then I would feel ashamed for eating and I would eat more, and then I would have proof that I was a terrible person and the cycle would go on and on, because when I felt fat and terrible I wouldn't want to go anywhere or see anyone so I would have to think of more excuses and find more valid reasons as to why I was saying no!

So I began to say no without giving a reason. Then I would sit with the feelings that came up in me of being a 'bad friend' or whatever. Sometimes I would still turn to food but over time this happened less and less. I was honoring my own needs. I am a natural introvert, I am sensitive, I find large groups difficult. I enjoy seeing people for short periods of time for deliciously deep conversations. After a beautiful connection with friends I like to retreat back to being with myself and my books. We are all different. We are allowed to be different. We are allowed to say 'no' and love ourselves and value our needs.

Bill of rights

I have the right to be treated with respect as an intelligent, capable and equal human being.

I have the right to have and express my own feelings and opinions.

I have the right to be listened to and taken seriously.

I have the right to set my own personal priorities.

I have the right to say NO without feeling guilty.

I have the right to ask for what I want.

I have the right to have my needs treated as being as important as the needs of others.

I have the right to make mistakes.

I have the right to change my mind.

I have the right to decline responsibility for other people's problems.

I have the right to say 'I don't understand' and ask for more information.

I have the right to deal with others without being dependent on them for approval.

I have the right to choose not to assert myself.

~ Anonymous

My heart-space is far more open now, I know I have no need to lie or make up excuses; I can be honest from my soul. If someone asks me to do something and I say 'no' I am still loving them from my heart. They may, or may not, feel that love but what they think of me is none of my business. If I know I am fearlessly and openly, loving them and myself, then my heart is at peace. We don't have to physically put ourselves in situations with people who we find difficult or draining. It is ok to have physical boundaries. Let the love flow anyway, there are no boundaries to love. Even if we really dislike someone we can let the love flow, we wish them no physical pain or harm and we can hope they find their own inner peace. Let the love flow.

The friends who left my life are still in my heart. Sometimes I feel sad, angry or bitter about the fact they no longer wish to speak to me BUT I also know I love them and wish them well and that I have forgiven myself, and them, for any past concerns between us. I let go, a lot. When feelings come up. I let go. If I feel my heart constrict, I breathe into it and I let go. I open myself out to the world because love is life.

Rambunctious resources for the exploration of assertiveness skills

♥ Boundaries, the importance of valuing yourself.
http://www.selfgrowth.com/articles/Boundaries_the_
importance.html.
♥ Anne Katherine. *Where to Draw the Line: How to Set Healthy Boundaries Every Day.*
♥ Cheryl Richardson. *Let me disappoint you. Sometimes it is ok to say no.*
http://www.healyourlife.com/author-cheryl-richardson
/2012/06/wisdom/personal-growth/let-me-disappoint-you

Chapter 13

Learning to self-soothe without food

Now that we have looked at thoughts and feelings and how to name and allow them safely we can begin to investigate learning how to self-soothe without food. Each individual will find their own personal recipe for self-soothing. It is about creating a toolkit for yourself so that you have alternative coping mechanisms to eating.

🖉 Take time to experiment and investigate what makes you feel better or calmer when things start to feel overwhelming. Remember that first and foremost you need to allow the feelings to come up, notice them, journal about them and then think about what would be soothing. Some ideas might include the following. Write your own list of lovely, nourishing strategies.

- Going for a walk in nature, alone or with a friend;
- Putting on soothing music and relaxing, or energetic music and dancing;
- Going to visit your favorite art gallery or museum;
- Looking at photographs that you treasure;
- Lying on the grass watching the clouds;
- Stroking a cat or dog;
- Taking a special, relaxing bath with candles and oils;
- Sitting all cuddled up on the sofa with a soft blanket and a warm drink;
- Getting a massage;
- Phoning a trusted friend;
- Reading a calming or inspiring book;
- Journaling;
- Do something creative – creativity feeds us. Draw, paint,

knit, sew or write. Explore creativity online. Creativity is a big outlet for feelings and thoughts;
- Meditate or listen to a relaxation CD;
- Clear out a cupboard that you have been meaning to clear;
- Take a nap;
- Read and write some positive affirmations.

Sometimes nothing will seem to work and you may well turn to food, remember this is normal. It is OK and it is safe. At these times it is important not to beat yourself up mentally about the behavior. Stay aware, acknowledge that you are eating for comfort. Eat mindfully taking time to taste and smell the food.

Reduce overwhelm and stress

Part of your toolkit is to recognize that stress and overwhelm can often trigger emotional eating. Each one of us will be stressed or overwhelmed by different things. You need to check in with yourself throughout the day to see how you are feeling. Learn about yourself. My own feelings of overwhelm (a big trigger for my emotional eating) get triggered when I see my to-do list full of projects like 'create website' or 'write book;' these are PROJECTS and not tasks, I know that in order to cope and not get overwhelmed I need to break the projects down into TASKS and not push myself to complete them in unrealistic timescales!

Find ways that help you to prevent stress and overwhelm, for example:

- Take a break from whatever you are working on each hour, even if it is just to walk to the ladies' room and stretch your legs!
- Write about how you feel;
- Turn your phone and computer off at 8pm so that you have time to unwind before bed;
- Listen to a relaxation CD at lunchtime or whenever is

going to be most helpful for you;

- Do 15 minutes of cleaning each day so that it doesn't stack up and become a huge task;
- Take breaks to meditate or walk;
- Slow down;
- Say 'no;'
- Breathe consciously and count your breath from one to ten and then back down again.

✎ What would help you to reduce stress and overwhelm in your life?

What you can do if the urge to eat becomes strong

First of all stop and breathe. You are feeling sensations and thinking thoughts and your unconscious mind is telling you to run to food. Stopping to breathe creates a loving gap between the thought/feeling/emotion and eating. This gap is precious. This gap represents awareness, it is compassionate and it helps you to become fully conscious.

Follow your breathing for a minute or two and be aware of the thoughts. Let them come up and realize they are just thoughts. Take a few more breaths and see if you can get in touch with your feelings, the deeper feelings below the initial 'I need to eat' feeling. Are you stressed? Overwhelmed? Sad? Happy? Notice the feeling and the sensations in your body. Be non-judgmental as you do this, just notice with curiosity. You might want to write about what you feel/think in your journal.

Next, ask yourself, 'what do I need?' You might need – a break, a walk, a rest, a hug, a chat with someone – really allow those needs to come up and honor them.

If after pausing and breathing and checking in you still want to eat, then do so mindfully. Say out loud or internally to yourself that you are making a conscious choice to cope with a situation by eating. Be compassionate with yourself; give yourself permission to eat without guilt, judgment or shame. It is OK to choose to eat. It does not make you a 'bad person.' Choose what you are going to eat, put it on a plate and go and sit down. Don't just think about sitting down and eating mindfully as you stand at the cupboard and put the food in your mouth. Taste the food, notice the texture. Notice also any thoughts/feelings that might come up. Write about it in your journal.

A tip that you might find really helpful when beginning self-exploration is to put post-it notes on the kitchen cupboards and refrigerator that say things like 'BREATHE & BE AWARE,' 'LOVE YOURSELF,' 'HOW DO YOU FEEL?,' 'WHAT DO YOU NEED?' This can help prevent an unconscious eating episode. Do this and see if it helps you, don't just think about it and think it might be a good idea. Actually go out and buy some post-it notes. We often read tips and think that they sound great but then never follow through with them. It is as though our mind is telling us that just reading the tip is enough! Play with the ideas presented in this book – some will feel nourishing to you and others won't, but take time to explore!

Rambunctious resources for the exploration of self-soothing

♥ All books by SARK can really feel the creative soul. SARK writes a lot about her own journey in life and how she takes care of herself with creativity.
http://planetsark.com
♥ Julia Cameron. *The Artist's Way.*
♥ Kris Carr.
http://crazysexylife.com
♥ Louise Hay. *You can heal your life.*
♥ Cheryl Richardson. *The art of extreme self care.*

Chapter 14

The power of gratitude, optimism and forgiveness

In the self-love chapter, we looked into some commitments that might be useful on the self-love journey. One of these was to keep a daily gratitude list. Here I am asking you to extend that. Each day, write ten things that you feel grateful for and ten things you feel proud about. Yes, proud. As mentioned earlier we rarely celebrate ourselves but it is so important!

🖉 Your journal is a safe place for celebration. Begin the daily habit of writing gratitude and celebration lists.

'Gratitude unlocks the fullness of life. It turns what we have into enough, and more. It turns denial into acceptance, chaos to order, confusion to clarity. It can turn a meal into a feast, a house into a home, a stranger into a friend.'
~ Melody Beattie

Here is a bit from my list:

Today I feel grateful for waking up in my warm cozy bed, for my loving husband and for my gorgeous dog, Freddy. I am grateful that I didn't miss the postman who had a package for me. I am also grateful that the sun shone and Freddy and I could have a lovely walk in the green field. Ooooh, there are so many things to be grateful for. I feel proud that I sat down to write even though I felt resistance! I also feel proud that I did some work on my website and managed to cook a lovely dinner from minimal ingredients!

✏ What are you grateful for and proud of today? Check in with your feelings and thoughts as you do this exercise – do you notice the critical voice or the saboteur getting in the way or are you just loving finding so many things to celebrate in your life?!

This exercise isn't just a bit of fun. It can be part of the healing journey and is a very powerful process. The relationship between our thoughts and our biology (or health of our body cells) entered the mainstream when Dr Bruce Lipton published *The biology of belief* in 2005. Scientific studies looking at optimism, gratitude and forgiveness and their impact on health are increasing in number. One scientific research paper [1] found that '"spiritual" positive emotions like hope, faith, forgiveness, joy, compassion and gratitude are extremely important in the relief of stress.' In the paper the author talks about the feel good 'love' hormone oxytocin – if we can cultivate the positive emotions just mentioned then oxytocin is likely to be produced in our bodies. Oxytocin seems to protect us against the negative impacts of fear, anxiety and depression such as high blood pressure and high levels of cortisol, a stress hormone. In fact oxytocin can help us to stay in a non-anxious state. Studies have also found that by soothing research subjects with videos of positive emotions (you can do it at home just by cuddling), you can lower pulse rate, speed heart recovery and enhance memory, creativity and social tolerance. Doing the opposite, by stimulating negative emotion, can reverse the process.

Gratitude has also been linked to wellbeing. Being grateful and keeping gratitude journals can help to treat stress and depression. Grateful people seem to have more positive ways of coping with the difficulties they experience in life, are more likely to seek support from other people and to reinterpret and grow from difficult experiences. Grateful people also seem to have less negative coping strategies, being less likely to try to avoid the problem, deny there is a problem, blame themselves, or cope through substance use.

Individuals who keep a daily gratitude journal seem to be more optimistic about life, more likely to exercise regularly, and felt better physically compared to those who recorded hassles or neutral life events.

Some ways to cultivate gratitude:

- Keep a daily gratitude journal;
- Think about a living person for whom you are grateful;
- Write about someone for whom you are grateful;
- Write a gratitude letter to deliver to someone;
- Write out positive affirmations such as,'I am filled with gratitude for the un-ending gifts that life gives me;'
- Look non-judgmentally at your thoughts to see where you are being overly negative and see if you can work on those areas.

Often thoughts stream through our minds and we don't notice their context. Keeping the gratitude list helps to focus us back to things that have been good that day. It is a great idea to set aside little mini-quiet times during the day when you can stop and breathe for two to five minutes and get back in touch with your centre and dis-identify from your thoughts.

Be grateful for yourself, your gifts, and your love. Celebrate your beautiful self.

'Gratitude gladdens the heart. It is not sentimental, not jealous, nor judgmental. Gratitude does not envy or compare. Gratitude receives in wonder the myriad offerings of the rain and the earth, the care that supports every single life. As gratitude grows it gives rise to joy. We experience the courage to rejoice in our own good fortune and in the good fortune of others.'
~ Jack Kornfield

Optimism

Albert Einstein said, 'The world we have created is a product of our thinking. It cannot be changed without changing our thinking.' Optimism and positive thinking are powerful. Quantum physics has found that thought is energy – so what kind of energy do you want to put out in the world? Is your glass half empty or half full? Constantly allowing your thoughts to run riot about how you can never heal and you'll never be free from emotional eating is not going to motivate you. Negative thinking makes life difficult and grey and makes any task seem like a mountain to climb. Again it all comes down to change. If your tendency has always been to be a negative thinker then optimism is a muscle you can choose to build. Remember you can always fake it until you make it!

It is important to sit and allow feelings to come up, if sadness comes up then let it come up; you might need to have a good cry and really feel that. However, if your thoughts are constantly beating you up with negativity then you can sit and observe that and choose to change. Begin working with some positive affirmations: 'I deeply and completely love and accept myself,' 'it is SAFE to think positive thoughts,' 'it is safe to be positive,' 'I allow my positivity to shine,' 'I can achieve my goals one step at a time.'

Optimism could be good for the health of our heart

Back in 2009, a study about optimism in women was published 2; the researchers found that optimists live healthier and longer lives than pessimists. Researchers at University of Pittsburgh followed more than 100,000 women. Optimists were found to have lower rates of coronary heart disease compared to pessimists. Women who were optimistic, those who expect good rather than bad things to happen, were 14% less likely to die from any cause than pessimists and 30% less likely to die from heart disease after eight years of follow up in the study.

Optimists also were also less likely to have high blood pressure, diabetes or smoke cigarettes. The research team, led Dr. Hilary Tindle, also looked at women who were highly mistrustful of other people, a group they called 'cynically hostile,' and compared them with women who were more trusting. Women in the cynically hostile group tended to agree with questions such as, 'I've often had to take orders from someone who didn't know as much as I did,' or, 'it's safest to trust nobody.' This kind of thinking was shown to take a toll various health problems.

At the end of the day, optimism makes us feel good! Begin setting up new happiness and positivity habits; really look for the good in your life and in any situation. It's not that you have to lie about what is going on, but look at every situation from all angles; there is always something positive to take. Simply learning from mistakes is very positive and allows us to make more conscious, future choices. We can learn to be grateful for our mistakes, grateful for the learning.

✐ Journal about the following: Take a look at the friendships and people in your life – are they positive or negative? Have you fallen into a place where you sit around and only share your woes and never your happiness and positive experiences? Are those friendships and relationships healthy for you or do you need some boundaries? Can you set up a 'positivity circle' where you and your friends share positive stories and joy?

Gratitude and optimism can help pull us out of thoughts that can send us running to food for comfort and support. They really are powerful tools to work with.

Forgiveness

Much has been said and written about forgiveness as a tool toward healing. It really can help us to release years of pain.

Forgiveness begins with self-forgiveness. You may well be

eating because you believe you are a 'bad' person, because you have made mistakes – these mistakes might have been as simple as dropping a pint of milk. Then you feel terrible about the eating, which usually leads to more eating! You may well find yourself saying sorry for everything and then eating to numb the ensuing guilt and shame. You may also overcompensate, to try and cover your shame, by being 'the good girl' the pleaser who tries to do everything right. All of this is exhausting. Shining the light of awareness on your thoughts and feelings can be so helpful to see that you are not, and never have been, 'bad' at all. None of us are 'bad' even if we make mistakes. It is the inner voice of the critic and saboteur that would have us believe we are bad. Sitting, being aware of these thoughts and remembering that we are not our thoughts is so important.

Loving yourself means loving yourself even when you make mistakes! Forgiveness is loving by its very nature.

'When you forgive yourself you make peace with something you did or didn't do that you feel bad about. Though you can't change what happened in the past you can lovingly take responsibility for your mistakes, make amends if possible, and make a sincere effort not to repeat the behavior in the future.'
~ Marci Shimoff

We need to stop judging ourselves, and start loving all of who we are. Be gentle when you make what you think is a mistake. Forgive yourself. Say something kind to yourself. 'I am willing to forgive myself and I deeply and completely love and accept myself.' Forgive yourself for the torture you have inflicted on yourself with your words and thoughts. Forgive yourself and then you can begin to open up to the idea of forgiving others who you believe have hurt you. Believe and know that you are forgiven.

On my personal self-forgiveness journey learned about ho'oponopono; it is an ancient Hawaiian 'art'. One of the main processes is repeating this sentence/mantra: 'I love you, I'm sorry, please forgive me, thank you, I love you,' over and over again. It is said to have a 'clearing' effect on the mind and past, old, unnecessary memories. People have used this as a self-healing mantra and say it is a way of forgiving ourselves (and others) and falling more deeply in love with the true goodness of who we are.

We are all human and we make mistakes. Sometimes we don't even realize what we are doing to ourselves until after the event and that is when self-compassion and self forgiveness are so important. So, forgive yourself today and make self-forgiveness, rather than beating up on yourself, a habit.

When we begin to forgive others, we need to remember that it doesn't mean that we were not hurt or that the person is 'getting away with it' or that we have to let that person back into our lives. Forgiveness is an act of love because it sets us free. When we forgive, it opens the heart to love. Forgiveness is an important step in the process of exploring emotional eating.

'Forgiving someone doesn't mean you have to hang out with them, it just means they don't have to hang out in your head.'
~ The global love project

If you have been through some very challenging experiences, you might want to work with a therapist or counselor before going straight into forgiveness. This would be an act of extreme self-love and a gift to yourself. I have experienced great healing through my therapy sessions in the past and have let go of a lot of past aches. In fact I have re-written my own negative stories, stories that I believed to be true, but they were subjective and only true when looking through one lens. Having a 360-degree view on a situation can really open life up!

'True forgiveness does not paper over what has happened in a superficial way. It is not a misguided effort to suppress or ignore our pain. It cannot be hurried. It is a deep process repeated over and over in our heart, which honors the grief and betrayal, and in its own time ripens into the freedom to truly forgive. Forgiveness does not forget nor does it condone the past. Forgiveness sees wisely. It willingly acknowledges what is unjust, harmful, and wrong. It bravely recognizes the sufferings of the past, and understands the conditions that brought them about. There is a strength to forgiveness.'
~ Jack Kornfield

✎ Begin with yourself. Journal about how you feel about forgiveness. Feel into your body and explore the sensations.

Be ultra gentle with yourself as you journey with forgiveness. Forgive yourself for emotionally eating. Eating to deal with emotions does not make you a bad person! It is an old coping mechanism, which you have been fearlessly and courageously exploring here. Have compassion for yourself and vow not to beat yourself up about your behavior any more. The light of compassion is healing beyond what we can conceive. If you had a daughter who ate to deal with her emotions would you beat her over the head with a stick and tell her she was bad and say nasty things to her? NO, you would love her as the precious child of the universe that she is, as you are. Love yourself like that. Do it today. Do it now.

Rambunctious resources for the exploration of gratitude, optimism and forgiveness

♥ SARK. *Glad no matter what. Transforming loss and change into gift and opportunity.*
   http://planetsark.com

♥ Louise Hay. *Give yourself permission to forgive.*
http://www.healyourlife.com/author-louise-l-hay/2012/07/
wisdom/inspiration/give-yourself-permission-to-forgive

♥ Marianne Williamson. *The Miracle of Forgiveness. Connecting back to spirit.*
http://www.healyourlife.com/author-marianne-williamson/
2012/05/wisdom/inspiration/the-miracle-of-forgiveness

♥ Esther and Jerry Hicks. *Ask and it is given.*

♥ Jack Kornfield. *The art of forgiveness, lovingkindness and peace.*

♥ For some meditations on Forgiveness visit Jack Kornfield's website:
http://www.jackkornfield.com

♥ Action for happiness.
http://www.actionforhappiness.org

Chapter 15

Food wisdom

This section has the potential to be vast. As a registered nutritionist with a passion for evidence based advice and a real love of good food I could write an entire book on food and emotional eating (and perhaps one day I will). Here, I have decided to include some main points and key issues because exploring emotional eating isn't really about food, although, as you will see, certain food choices can impact emotional eating – so it IS about the food too! What I want to make clear is that this section is not about dieting, weight loss or calories. It is about learning how food can impact mood and how mood can impact food choice.

You might think that when you are emotional you decide to eat food – which is true – BUT certain foods can impact your body chemistry, which can lead to cravings and more food being eaten. Some food can also impact the mood, which can lead to more emotional eating because you feel emotional! A vicious circle is created that can self-perpetuate further eating.

In the next few pages I will be taking some time to share some of my knowledge about empowered food choice. It is important to remember that we are not talking about dieting. This is about learning food wisdom and learning that sometimes our food choices can actually negatively impact our moods. At the same time some foods can help improve the mood, which can definitely be empowering!

If you decide you would like some more specific help in the area of food choice then I suggest you book a Support Session with me (or a registered nutritionist with a specialism in the area of emotional eating) where we can work together on your own personal eating patterns and how they might be impacting your emotional eating.

Stress and food choice

As we have explored, often when we are stressed and overwhelmed we often turn to eating. We have looked at ways to interrupt the cycle by being aware of our thoughts and feelings and seeing if there is anything we need in terms of support or taking time to relax etc. This is important. Implementing steps to reduce stress helps us to make more empowered choices and we find we turn to food less.

There are other important reasons why it is a good idea to reduce stress levels. Stress and depression have actually been found to influence our food choices. Stress tends to make us choose less healthy food options, which are often high in sugary carbohydrates and low in vegetables and fruits. These less healthy choices can then impact our blood sugar levels (which I will discuss later), which causes us to crave more sugar, sugary foods also put further stress on the body – so you can see how a cycle is set up. We think we are 'bad' for all this eating we are doing but actually the biological changes going on in our body make it quite difficult to pull out of the cycle. I mention this so that you might feel empowered to keep health-full foods in your cupboards and make wise choices when you turn to food in order to prevent this cycles from being set up and causing you emotional distress.

Long-term stress can lead to something known as adrenal depletion. The adrenal glands sit above the kidneys and they produce stress hormones such as cortisol and adrenaline. When we have been overwhelmed and stressed for a long period of time these adrenal glands get tired and don't work optimally. When this happens we can experience low energy, poor concentration, poor mood, food cravings and insomnia. Long term stress can often cause depletion of B-vitamins, magnesium, zinc and vitamin C because these nutrients are needed for healthy adrenal gland function.

So you can see how important stress management is on the

journey toward healing from emotional eating. As well as relaxation techniques, massage, journaling, mindfulness, self-love and self-care as discussed earlier, a healthful delicious diet, rich in vegetables, fruits, nuts, omega 3 fats and other unprocessed foods is definitely beneficial.

Nutrient density – empowered food choice doesn't have to be boring

Nutrient dense food is food that is raucously rich in vitamins, minerals, fiber, essential fats and plant chemicals known as phytonutrients, which protect our cells and are important for health. I call these foods 'love superfoods.' Healthful eating can impact every area in the body, can protect against cancer, heart disease, osteoporosis, depression and much more. Healthful eating is self-love.

Foods that are processed and 'white or beige' are empty foods, eating these foods does not nourish us or nurture us. These foods provide us with very limited vitamins and minerals and often make us feel hungry and wanting more and sometimes they can lead to poor mood. Nutrient dense foods tend to make us feel full and satisfied and can actually boost our mood.

Examples of nutrient dense foods include – vegetables, salad vegetables and leafy greens, fruits (especially berries like strawberries, blueberries, cherries and raspberries), beans/pulses, wholegrains, oily fish, nuts and seeds, avocadoes, sweet potatoes. Variety really is the spice of life – there are so many delicious healthful foods to choose.

Blood sugar balance, mood and cravings

Foods which are high in carbohydrate (sugars and starches) e.g. sugar, potatoes, bread, grains, biscuits, cakes, pasta and rice are broken down in the body to form glucose (a form of sugar), which is then absorbed into the blood stream to provide fuel/energy for the body. Glucose is the simplest form of sugar and main source of energy for our body cells including brain cells. We need enough glucose in the blood to provide energy but too much can damage our cells by causing inflammation in the body.

Our body needs to have balanced blood sugar levels for physical and mental wellbeing. Imbalances in blood sugar levels during the day can lead to the following symptoms:

- Fluctuating energy levels and fatigue/tiredness;
- Low energy in the mid-afternoon;
- Poor energy levels in the morning;
- Poor concentration;
- Irritability;
- Mood swings;
- Depression;
- Forgetfulness;
- Dizziness;
- Food Cravings;
- Increased appetite;
- Insomnia;
- Excess thirst;
- Complex interactions between insulin and fat cells that can lead to fat being stored.

A brief overview of how blood sugar levels can be disrupted: our blood sugar levels increase which causes the pancreas to produce insulin. Insulin is vital as it allows glucose to enter our cells where it is used to provide us with energy for all body processes (pretty crucial huh?!). As the glucose enters our cells our blood sugar levels return to normal. If a meal is eaten that is rich in carbohydrate foods, especially ones that release their sugar quickly (known as high GI or glycaemic index foods – which we will come on to later), and lacking in protein and essential fats (which help to prevent blood sugar spikes), e.g. sugary breakfast cereals, white rice, white pasta, biscuits, then the carbohydrates are rapidly digested and lots of glucose is released very quickly into the blood. Blood sugar levels rise rapidly – this causes the body to react really quickly to produce too much insulin, which causes the glucose to leave the blood quickly – this often leads to a huge dip in blood sugar levels. When blood sugar gets too low we can experience many of the symptoms listed above and since the body cannot function with such low blood sugar levels we often reach for more sugary food, leading to a blood sugar roller-coaster and many unpleasant symptoms, which can seem distressing!

Before getting on to looking at how best to eat to balance blood sugar a few other factors, which negatively impact the blood sugar balance, need to be mentioned:

Tea, coffee, cigarettes and fizzy drinks – these can rapidly raise blood sugar levels. They contain chemicals such as caffeine and nicotine, which are stimulants. Alcohol is also a stimulant which impacts our blood sugar levels in a way that can lead to cravings and mood imbalances. Artificial sweeteners are also stimulants and can impact the mood; they are NOT a healthful, loving option for the body.

As we have previously learned – stress also interferes with blood sugar balance, so often stressed individuals will crave sugary carbohydrates.

Empowered eating to keep blood sugar levels beautifully balanced

- Reduce intakes of stimulants such as tea, coffee and cigarettes. If you do want to drink caffeinated drinks make sure you do so with food that contains proteins and slow release carbohydrates. Try not to drink caffeine on its own.
- Even decaffeinated coffee contains stimulants. Herbal tea, redbush tea or coffee substitutes are a good choice.

- Reduce refined carbohydrates such as sugar, white flour products, sweets, biscuits and white rice.
- Eat 'slow release' (low GI – they release sugar slowly) carbohydrates which are wholegrain e.g. oats, millet, quinoa, wholegrain basmati rice.
- Snack on a few nuts not cereal bars.
- Never skip breakfast.
- Don't skip meals – it really impacts the blood sugar and can lead to huge cravings and problems with mood.
- Eat small frequent meals during the day.
- Include protein with every meal (we will look at this later but protein helps to prevent blood sugar imbalance).
- Dried fruit and fruit juices rapidly raise blood sugar so limit these to 1-2 times per day and eat with a meal that contains protein.
- Vegetables are a great source of slow release carbohydrate and they are also nutrient dense, rich in vitamins, minerals and fiber. Vegetables with hummus or a bean dip makes a great snack.
- Reduce alcohol intake and if you are drinking do it with a meal to minimize the impact on blood sugar levels.
- Movement can help the body use insulin more efficiently.
- Reduce stress as much as possible.

Glycaemic Index or GI

GI is a system of classification, or ranking, that is given to carbo-hydrate foods depending on how they affect our bodily blood sugar levels. A low GI food or meal takes a longer time to release sugar into the bloodstream. A high GI food or meal releases sugar very quickly into the bloodstream. Adding protein and essential fats to a meal help to reduce the GI of the meal and helps us to balance our blood sugar levels.

Examples of low GI carbohydrate foods that release sugar slowly: pulses such as lentils, chickpeas, kidney beans and butterbeans. Apples, plums, cherries, blueberries, raspberries, grapefruit, peas, avocado, courgette/zucchini, spinach, peppers, onions, mushrooms, leafy greens, beans, sprouts, mange tout, cauliflower, broccoli, unsweetened yoghurt, milk, nuts.

Examples of medium GI foods: sweet potatoes, new potatoes, carrots, sweetcorn, peas, wholegrain pasta, oats, wholegrain rye bread, buckwheat, bulgar wheat, brown rice, grapes, oranges, kiwi fruits, mango, beetroot, fresh dates, figs.

Examples of high GI foods which release sugar rapidly into the bloodstream: sugar, glucose, high fructose corn syrup, honey, pineapple, ripe banana, raisins, baked potatoes, rice cakes, couscous, cornflakes, muffins, biscuits, cakes, crumpets, refined foods, cream crackers.

We do not need to ban all high GI foods from our eating, we just need to be aware that they can disrupt the blood sugar and can lead to cravings and mood imbalances. Including high GI foods as part of a meal that includes protein and essential fats will help to keep the blood sugar balanced.

To check the GI of foods online the best resource is this one at the University of Sydney: http://www.glycemicindex.com.

Powerful Protein

Protein is important for many reasons; it provides the building blocks (amino acids) for repair of the body and is important for the structure of bone, skin, hair and our internal organs. It is vital for the immune system and is used to make hormones.

Good sources of protein include unprocessed meat, unprocessed fish, eggs, hemp seeds, beans, lentils, pulses, quinoa, nuts and seeds.

In terms of emotional eating, protein is important to know about because it is used by the body to make certain brain chemicals, known neurotransmitters, and it also helps to keep us feeling fuller for longer as well as helping to balance blood sugar levels.

Protein is essential for healthy neurotransmitter (brain chemical) balance – this has a vital impact on our moods. You may have heard of the natural feel-good chemicals in the brain such as serotonin, dopamine and endorphins? Protein is used to make these so it is important to get enough. If our serotonin levels are low we can experience low mood, sleep issues, tiredness and gut symptoms as well as food cravings. Stress, refined carbohydrates, alcohol and drugs can also interfere with the production of natural neurotransmitters in the brain.

Plan to eat protein as a part of every meal and snack – it will help to keep you feeling full, aid blood sugar balance and keeps the mood stabilized, it might also help to prevent cravings.

Fat can be fabulous

Fat is not evil and it doesn't make us fat. The old horror stories about fat were a big fat lie. The fats in processed foods, known as trans fats or hydrogenated fat, are definitely not good kinds of fat; they have been linked to certain kinds of cancers and heart problems. However, some fats are essential – they are called essential fats because they cannot be made in the body, which means we have to get them from our food. Without them the body cannot function properly. The fats found in nuts, seeds, avocados, olive oil and especially oily fish are really important for the body.

Omega 3 fatty acids (specifically the long chain ones known as EPA and DHA) are my big interest and I studied and researched them for a long while (and I still do). These omega 3 fats are found in oily fish such as salmon, mackerel, trout and sardines. I have been particularly interested in how these fats are vital for the function of the brain and can help reduce the risk of depression and other mood problems as well as having an impact on regulating food cravings and appetite.

Here are a few reasons why omega 3 fats are so vital for the body and brain:

- Provide the raw material from which many hormones are made;
- Vital for the correct function of the brain, lack of omega 3 fats is implicated in depression and low mood;
- Vital for the nervous system, immune system and cardio-vascular system (heart and circulation);
- Important for the heart and linked to a reduced risk of cancer;
- Important for the skin;
- Helps the absorption of certain vitamins;
- Can help to manage Premenstrual Syndrome, PMS, since it is vital for hormone production;
- Has been shown to reduce food cravings and can regulate the appetite.

Eating two portions of oily fish every week is a good way to ensure you are getting your omega 3s. However many people don't eat oily fish twice every single week and if you suffer from low mood or high stress it might be that you need more than this. In this case you might want to consider a fish oil supplement. If you want to discuss this with me then please book a Butterfly Love Support Session (details in the resources section).

What about vegetarians and vegans?

This is a really important question. Short chain omega 3 fats can be found in flaxseeds and some green leafy vegetables and hemp seeds. The problem is that the body finds it really hard to convert these into the longer versions which are found in fish and a vegetarian/vegan would need to make sure that they included a lot of these short chain fats into their daily diet. However, there is some great news – there is now a really good Vegan supplement made from algae that contains the long chain EPA and DHA fats. It is called opti3, you can find out about this at www.opti3omega.com.

Fiber

Fiber is important to mention because it can help us to feel fuller for longer and has an impact on our satiety. It is also really important for the health of our digestive system.

There are two types of fiber:

Soluble fiber – found in oats, rye, barley, pulses, beans, apples and citrus fruit;

Insoluble fiber – from the cellulose of plant walls, found in vegetables and some grains.

Eating gorgeous, health-full foods such as wholegrains, lentils, beans, pulses, fruits, vegetables, nuts and seeds will provide plentiful amounts of funky fiber for your fabulous body!

Vibrant Vitamins and Miraculous Minerals

An entire encyclopedia about vitamins and minerals, as well as associated plant compounds known as bioflavonoids, could be written but it is not important here to get bogged down in too much information. What is important to know is for the body to function at its best, to function optimally, it is crucial that we eat high quality, nutrient dense, foods which are packed with vitamins and minerals.

As I mentioned earlier, stress can increase our need for certain vitamins and minerals so eating food that packs a big nutrient punch can help us stay well and happy.

The key points are:

• Eat a VARIETY of colorful fruits and vegetables, at least five portions per day (but aim for more, they taste and look so scrumptious). Don't stick to what you know, look at all the different vegetables and fruits available and don't be afraid to try new things. The internet is full of recipes so if you don't know what to do with a certain vegetable or fruit

then Google it!
- Eat wholegrains– oats, rye, quinoa, millet, basmati rice.
- Eat unprocessed meat and fish.
- Nuts and seeds are packed with minerals and fiber as well as certain vitamins. Make sure you buy the unsalted ones with their skins still on.
- Include beans and pulses (such as lentils and chickpeas) into your cooking.

When you eat and choose food do so from a place of extreme self-love. Listen to your inner wisdom, choose food from the heart, nourishing, nurturing foods.

Key points about food wisdom and a few meal and snack ideas

- Food is nourishing and is vital for your body to function well. Try to think of food as medicine and not just in terms of dieting or weight loss.
- Use the food wisdoms and be wise when you choose.

There are some high profile advisors who suggest that when you feel like going to eat you should check in with yourself and see what it is that you are drawn to eating. In some respects I totally agree, we can listen to what is going on with us and then eat mindfully. There is also a problem with this method e.g. let's say you decide you would really love a chocolate biscuit because it's chocolatey and crunchy and sweet and a bit salty at the same time. Perhaps a childlike part of you wants this because you were not allowed chocolate biscuits as a child, or they were restricted. You can choose the biscuit and sit and eat it mindfully as we have discussed. HOWEVER this could well lead to your blood sugar becoming imbalanced and then you feel drawn to eat more and more sweet or carbohydrate foods and before you know it you are doing more than emotionally eating, you are on a blood sugar rollercoaster. My suggestion is that if you decide to choose a chocolate biscuit then do so, but also (be a good parent to yourself and) eat a few unsalted nuts (e.g. four to eight) or some seeds (about a dessertspoon). The fiber, protein and good fats in these will help to keep your blood sugar levels stable. (I discuss this further in the next section).

A word on nutrient supplements

Supplements should never be considered as an alternative to a healthy diet but they can be very useful. I certainly take supplements but as a registered nutritionist I know which supplements are of a high quality and also what dosages to take. It is never a good idea to self-prescribe supplements, it is always a good idea to check with a medical doctor or a registered nutritionist first. It is especially important to check with a health professional if you are already taking prescribed medications and certain supplements can interfere with these.

- Do not skip meals and always eat breakfast.
  Eating a snack between breakfast and lunch and between lunch and dinner can also help to stabilize your blood sugar.

- Balance your blood sugar to help prevent cravings and binges.
  Include protein with every meal and snack. Include slow release (low GI) carbohydrates into your meal and plenty of vegetables. Minimize sugar and refined, quick release (high GI) carbohydrates as well as caffeine, alcohol and artificial sweeteners.

- Including plenty of fresh vegetables, fruits, slow release wholegrains, unprocessed quality proteins, beans, pulses, nuts, seeds and essential omega 3 fats will help to make sure your body is getting what it needs.

- Make food interesting.
  Use olive oil, garlic, lemon, herbs and spices in your cooking to add flavor and vibrancy for the tongue!

- VARIETY – eat different foods.
  Don't get stuck in a routine with food, get lots of color, texture and flavor from trying all kinds of different foods. Routines and controls are very rigid. We are interested in loosening our control and becoming freer. The ideas below are just that – IDEAS – this is not a 'meal plan' these are just a few simple ideas. You can use some of these ideas and also listen to your own body wisdom when it comes to food choice.

The following are a few ideas – this is not a diet plan for you to follow. Use your inner wisdom. Tune in to your Wise Self when making food choices. Eat what is succulent, delicious and nourishing for your soul. Let go of rigidity. Don't let the inner child part of you call the shots. Listen beyond and hear the wisdom of your body. It can take time to hear that wisdom. It can take time to learn what the body wants and needs. As you begin to listen and tune in your palate and tastes may well change, you might catch yourself craving a crisp salad, a smoothie, a vegetable juice, some homemade soup or roast butternut squash. You may feel called to savor the taste and texture of a banana or crunchy carrot. Perhaps you'll want to bake a cake from scratch and experiment using dried fruit instead of refined sugar and ground almonds in place of white flour. Listen in. It might be that you need a walk, a hug or a rest and not food at all. Let yourself 'be' and you'll soon hear.

Bright and breezy breakfast ideas:

- Oats with seeds, nuts and a few dried dates or a banana for sweetness. Use hot or cold milk or milk alternatives such as hemp, almond, or coconut milk;
- Mixed berry smoothie blended with nuts and seeds – add some coconut milk or yoghurt if you like;
- Cottage cheese with fresh fruit and sunflower seeds;
- Scrambled egg with mushrooms, peppers and tomatoes (or made into an omelet);
- Wholegrain rye toast with almond butter;
- Plain yoghurt with nuts, seeds and berries.

Lovely lunches:

- Large bowl of salad leaves with an olive oil and balsamic vinegar dressing – with tuna or eggs and a few oatcakes;
- Vegetable soup with beans/pulses or some chicken with oatcakes or rye bread;
- Mixed bean salad with fresh leaves;
- Baked sweet potato with salad, cottage cheese or tuna;
- Rye bread sandwich with avocado and tahini (sesame seed paste) used as a spread;
- Vegetable omelet with salad;
- Rice and lentil salad with lots of green, leafy vegetables and an olive oil and balsamic dressing.

Delicious dinners:

- Salmon (trout, sardines or mackerel) with new potatoes, broccoli and a mixed salad;
- Vegetable curry with lentils and wholegrain basmati rice;
- Nut roast with roast squash/pumpkin, broccoli and a side salad;

- Baked sweet potato with hummus, kale and peas;
- Grilled chicken with roast Mediterranean vegetables and quinoa;
- Lentil and chickpea loaf with a large mixed salad;
- Chili made with lean beef mince, turkey mince or mixed pulses, include plenty of vegetables in the chili such as peppers, courgette and aubergine/eggplant, served with wholegrain basmati rice.

Scrumptious snacks:

- Oat cakes or rye bread with guacamole, lentil pate, hummus, tahini or nut spread;
- Vegetable sticks e.g. cucumber, carrot, celery with guacamole, lentil pate, hummus, tahini or nut spread;
- A small handful (about 25-30g) of unsalted nuts e.g. Brazil nuts, almonds, walnuts, hazelnuts, cashew nuts;
- A tablespoon of seeds e.g. sunflower, pumpkin, hemp;
- A cup of berries with a tablespoon of seeds or some nuts;
- Unsweetened natural yoghurt with fruit;
- Raw, dark chocolate (a small piece 20-25g) with a dessert spoon of seeds or a few nuts.

There are plenty of amazing recipe books full of delicious, nutritious, health-full ideas for meals; I have listed some books in the resources section at the end of the chapter.

Many books on compulsive eating advocate the non-diet approach and the 'legalization' of foods that the individual has previously labeled off limits. I agree with this approach to some extent in the sense that we need to stop labeling ourselves as 'bad' if we eat foods, which are not necessarily highly nutritious. However, I am an advocate of health, not diets but health, and I am a passionate and dedicated registered nutritionist. As mentioned, some foods, especially those high in sugars and quick release carbohydrates, can trigger binges for some people due to the blood sugar imbalances they can create. I certainly do not suggest deprivation or any kind of food banning – but I do suggest food wisdoms. I also suggest that prior to making a food choice we shine the light of self-awareness onto our eating. We stop to ask how we feel, what we need. We select some food and make sure we have protein present and we eat mindfully, tasting every bite and not inhaling large quantities of foods in an unconscious manner (although if this happens we need to practice self-forgiveness and self-love and compassion and not think we are 'bad').

For example, if you really want a carbohydrate-rich snack or some milky-sweet chocolate – then allow yourself a portion. Put it on a plate. Be aware that it can impact the body blood sugar and hence the mood and further cravings. Choose some protein-rich food and put that on the plate too, knowing it will help to minimize blood sugar imbalances and perhaps prevent a binge.

Before eating anything we need to stop and breathe and get in touch with ourselves, making the food choice from a place of peace and awareness. Food really can impact us in a physiological/biological way. What we eat does matter – for our health, our mood, our wellbeing. If we eat something that triggers our body chemistry to change and we start craving things then we might binge even if we are loving ourselves deeply, simply because of the stuff going on in the body.

As a registered nutritionist with vast knowledge and passion for health I simply cannot advocate an 'eat what you desire' approach. After years of dieting your taste may have changed and psychological attachments to certain foods may have been developed; in addition to this your metabolism might be out of whack, so time and patience is needed with food. The child within you might want to eat foods that were forbidden to you in childhood – and that's ok, we can allow for that, but at the same time we need to be the loving parent with the wisdom to allow a moderate amount of the previously forbidden food, together with some nutritious delights too. Over time you will realize that no food is 'forbidden' and that your desire for such foods slows right down. You may well find that these old binge-buddies taste too sweet, too artificial, too salty, and just not tasteful at all.

Love yourself as you find peace with food. Ask yourself what you would choose to eat if you really loved yourself in that moment – and if the answer is chocolate then eat the chocolate!!

Knowing when you're truly, physically hungry may take time. Choosing to feel a feeling rather than eat the feeling may also take time. Have compassion for yourself during this time. If you feel overwhelmed or sad and feel unable to sit with feelings and you choose to still eat food – do it mindfully and realize that it is a choice, don't be judgmental about that choice. Say to yourself, 'I feel overwhelmed right now and food feels like the only way to cope. I know that as time goes on I will find other ways to deal with the overwhelm but right now I am choosing food and that's ok. I deeply and completely love and accept myself.' Then sit down and eat the food mindfully.

Good food, really good food, tastes delicious. Become a fan of delicious tastes! Often the most nutritious, colorful foods taste the best. For example, recently I went to a raw-food restaurant and the food was so amazingly tasty, so much flavor. Food is also medicine, there is no room in this book to write about all I know about nutritional medicine but it is exciting. Food also impacts the brain and our moods that is why I cannot write, f*ck it, eat what you want' – because I love you and your body and want you to love it too.

Much of the food industry truly perplexes and angers me – they churn out nutritionally devoid stuff, which they call food. Some of their offerings are so unnecessary. Real food tastes great, the body loves it, and it doesn't set up unhealthy obsessions in the brain. It is a challenge to rise above some of the rubbish that is produced by the food industry, but when self-love is strongly in place it becomes easier to choose lovingly to feed the body.

Sleep impacts appetite and food choice

Are you exhausted and reaching for food in order to get an energy boost? Are you really hungry or just plain tired? Sleep is important for our bodies for so many reasons. One reason is that it seems to have an impact on our appetite. Aim for a minimum of seven hours. If we are well rested we will feel better mentally and more able to choose healthy lifestyle behaviors.

Sleep also impacts the hormones that regulate our appetite. Short sleep is associated with higher levels of the appetite-stimulating hormone ghrelin and lower levels of the appetite-sating hormone leptin. Too little sleep can also impact insulin – which has all kinds of impact on the body. Short sleep can mean higher levels of the stress hormone cortisol; too much cortisol can impact insulin too. Stress, as mentioned earlier can often have us reaching for food.

Tiredness can also cause us to reach for food in order to give us energy and when we are tired we often feel less inclined to move our bodies. If we are well rested we will feel better mentally, clearer and more able to choose healthy lifestyle behaviors compared to when we are sleep deprived and a bit foggy-headed.

Personally, I know that when I don't get good sleep I find my stress levels elevated and my coping strategies diminished. I also tend to become quite emotional and notice that my appetite is elevated. Getting good amounts of good quality sleep is a massive self-care priority for me. Turning off my phone and laptop before 8pm is a rule I do my best to stick to! It leaves me time to just be in peace with my journal and my books, getting into a really quiet and still space which makes sleep so much easier to slip into.

Can you make sleep a priority in your life? Switch the stimulating TV programs, phones and computers off for at least an hour before bed? Even committing to going to bed 20 minutes earlier could start to make a difference. Sleeping enough helps make our waking hours more pleasurable and more productive. Sleep needs to be part of your self-care and self-love routine.

Listen to the wisdom of your body

It is not more spiritual to eat healthy foods. You are not less spiritual if you eat a bit of chocolate. You are not a 'bad' person because of what you eat.

We are all as spiritual as one another. We are all whole pieces of the Divine. Ask yourself what you would eat if you loved yourself, truly. Do not compare your food choices to other peoples. It is not a competition.

Aim to taste things. Aim for unprocessed, real food. Check in with your feelings and needs first – can you soothe the feeling in a different way and then make a food choice? I am all for healthy food, natural, unprocessed food, but I am not for the obsession with food. Listen to your soul. Your soul feeds you and you feed your body. This YOU, is your True Nature, Divinity, It.

Too much 'healthy' isn't healthy! The aim here is not to switch to an obsession with healthy food, detoxing, cleansing or over-exercising. No. The reason for this book is to see that beneath all of our obsessing with food is a need or a feeling that wants our attention, our aim is to be able to allow that feeling and fulfill that need without trying to solve it or cover it with food – be that healthful food or not. Comforting ourselves with chocolate or with carrots is not the solution.

The other day I made myself a smoothie and I put in too many greens, it was way too bitter and tasted horrible but I caught myself drinking it anyway because:

1. It was good for me and...
2. I didn't want to waste it!

It wouldn't have been a waste to throw it out; I am not a human dustbin myself. I could also have stopped to add a banana to sweeten it out a bit. I didn't really think about it until I almost finished. Then I stopped and decided I'd had enough and laughed at myself for getting caught in that place again.

> 'When food is simply food, we do not need very much of it. On the other hand, when food is used to express how needy we feel and how bad we feel about needing so much, no portion is ever big enough.'
> ~ Jane Hirschmann & Carol Munter. *When women stop hating their bodies. Freeing yourself from food and weight obsession.*

Dieting really doesn't work for most people. Most individuals will gain the weight they have lost back within two years and possibly gain back more. There are so many studies now to show that diets just don't cut it. The way out is to let love in, love yourself first, choosing loving foods, let go of the obsessions and the control. Then begin to listen to your body. Know what hunger is again, don't eat by the clock. Check in with yourself. You don't have to eat certain foods at certain times either. Use your body wisdom not the outside cues from food industry, diet experts of well meaning friends and family. This will take time. We haven't listened to our bodies for so many years. Letting go of using food to cope with emotions is hard; it's like letting go of a friend. You have to learn to be that friend for yourself now and find authentic people to surround yourself with too.

Once you can begin to let go of the obsession with food and weight, your life will open up. You can begin to fall in love with yourself, with life, with your own potential. It is sad that so many women are stymied by the diet, body, shame world. It's just not ok. It might feel frightening to trust yourself after trusting the diet books for so long.

When you start checking in with your body and feeling the

sensations there, you might find that sometimes the hunger you thought was for food is actually a hunger to shine and no amount of eating can satisfy that. Your hunger might be for creativity, dance, writing, poetry, and gardening. We are here in the world to shine our own particular sparkle. Investigate this.

It can literally take years to re-train ourselves to feel safe enough to wait to eat until we are hungry. How often have you looked at the clock and just decided it was time to eat without checking in to see if you actually wanted to eat? That was definitely how I used to eat. Completely unconsciously, and I am not judging myself for that but that is how it was. The clock struck 12.45pm and I would decide it must be time for lunch.

For me, things changed out of a very painful situation. When my relationship broke down without warning I was plunged into real darkness and for two weeks I felt no hunger. None. I could barely eat. I went from almost constant grazing to eating minimal amounts. I also thought nothing about food. It didn't cross my mind, whereas before it was constantly on my mind. After two weeks I began to feel hunger and out of this tragic situation came healing for my deeper food wounds. I listened carefully to my body. I ate when I felt hunger and I ate what my body wanted and I was able to stop eating when I had enough. This had nothing to do with the clock. I found a rhythm. I honored myself. This process has also had an impact on my ability to be honest with people – sometimes when I am out I am not hungry when the people I am with are. I am happy to sit and have a drink whilst they eat. It is really amazing how sometimes they try to force me to eat because they are uncomfortable eating alone. Other times I am hungry when others are not and I am happy to pull some nuts out of my bag and have a munch. Being an early riser, my breakfast is often eaten before 7.30pm. At about 11am I often get hungry again, not for a snack but for something more substantial. So my main meal of the day is often around 11am. In the evenings I don't tend to get so hungry and might have a light meal at 5.30pm. My husband, on the other hand, has his main meal in the evening about 7pm and that is fine. We have communicated honestly about this, I sit with him whilst he eats and we chat and catch up with our news from the day. It works and I don't apologize for following my body rhythms and I don't try to force Chris to follow mine.

This kind of body rhythm with food may take time and experimentation. Give yourself that gift of exploration; begin to honor your body and the wisdom contained within it.

Consider keeping a food and feelings diary

For two to four weeks you might want to consider keeping a food and feelings diary. This can be particularly helpful if you feel that you are still 'going unconscious' and finding yourself eating without stopping to pause, breathe and be aware of your thoughts and feel into the sensations and emotions in your body.

It is important that the diary is not used as a mental base-ball bat! It is not a way to beat yourself up. It's all about learning what might be triggering you and bringing the light of awareness to your emotional eating. It is a gentle, loving and curious process.

Make sure that the notebook you use is small and portable (small enough to fit into your pocket). It doesn't need to be fancy, as you will be throwing it away once you have gained the insight you need. Carry it with you and each time you find yourself eating write down:

a) The time of day;

b) What it is that you are eating;

c) How you felt immediately before you ate;

d) Note down anything that might be useful like *I had loads of stressful emails *I had no time to stop and connect this morning *My mum is ill in hospital *I broke a plate *I was really excited about a letter I got in the post.

You can look at your diary at the end of the day and see what has been going on. This can be helpful to teach you about triggers and then you can put plans in place to prevent lapses from happening (we'll look at lapses next).

Things to look out for:

- Where is there stress, are you reacting to that stress with food?
- Are your food choices disrupting your blood sugar levels and impacting your cravings?
- Are there people in your life who are increasing your stress levels?
- Look for any clues and take them on board gently and with compassion.

Use the diary to remind you about pausing, stopping, checking in with thoughts and emotions, mindful eating and stress reduction. Be very gentle with yourself and completely non-judgmental!

Dealing with a lapse in a positive way

Never feel bad, or criticize yourself if you fall back into your emotional eating patterns:

- Re-frame the event in your mind – a lapse is not a disaster. It is a learning experience.
- Take time to sit peacefully with your breath and explore your thoughts and feelings. Write about it.
- Were you feeling stressed or anxious before you ate?
- Was there a need that you felt was unmet and so you turned to food?
- Did you have a difficult or negative conversation with someone?
- Did you eat something today that disrupted your blood

sugar levels?

- Can you see how you were led to emotional eating? It is great to see the triggers and high-risk situations because you can begin to plan how to notice them for next time.
- After you have sat and done a bit of exploration it is time to move forwards. You have learned from this experience.
- What can you do now to love yourself? Can you call a friend? Go for a walk? Look at your list of self-soothing activities and alternatives to eating. Do something ultra-nourishing for yourself. Do not sit and obsess about the episode.
- Do you need to get some support from a friend or counselor, or book a support session with me?
- Keep things in perspective. Focus on all of the positive changes that you have made. Journal about the positive changes. Find something about the lapse that feels like learning. Each time you emotionally eat is a learning opportunity and part of the process of change. If you hadn't accomplished something, there would be no 'lapse.' Perhaps you can even find something to be grateful for from this experience.
- Practice self-forgiveness and self-love.

Rambunctious resources for the exploration of food wisdom

♥ One-to-one Support Session with me (I am a registered nutritionist); check the website www.nurturewithlove.com or email me ani@nurturewithlove.com for more details.
♥ Dr Christiane Northrup. *Women's Bodies, Women's Wisdom. The complete guide to women's health and wellbeing.*
♥ Dr John Briffa. *Escape the Diet Trap.* www.drbriffa.com
♥ Professor Basant K. Puri and Hilary Boyd. *The natural way*

to beat depression. The groundbreaking discovery of EPA to change your life.

- ♥ Kris Carr.
  www.crazysexylife.com
- ♥ Food and behavior research.
  http://www.fabresearch.org/3
- ♥ Professor Basant K. Puri. *The natural energy cookbook.*
- ♥ Past articles I have written about Food and Mood:
  http://www.nurturewithlove.com/feed-your-brain-and-improve-your-mood.
- ♥ This is a fantastic leaflet written by the Mental Health Foundation:
  http://www.mentalhealth.org.uk/publications/healthy-eating-depression/ – it is free to download.
- ♥ Karlyn Grimes. *The everything anti-inflammation diet book.*
- ♥ Ani Phyo. *Ani's raw food kitchen.*
- ♥ Barbara Cousins. *Vegetarian cooking without. Recipes free from added gluten, sugar, yeast, dairy products, meat, fish, saturated fat.*

Chapter 16

Marvelous movement and being in your precious body

Earlier we investigated our thinking and looked at how we tend to be 'unconscious walking heads,' always in our thoughts, turning things over in our minds. Exploration through awareness of these thoughts is a great step, as is exploration of feelings and sensations in the body.

The next step is to take focused time each week for movement; this does not mean obsessive exercise with a focus on calorie burning. Moving the body, breathing in the awareness of being in a body and not just in our head is really important.

Movement could be:

- Walking, consciously, feeling our feet on the ground, focusing on the breath and the movement of the body and letting go of thought;
- Walking with a friend;
- Swimming;
- Trying out a new dance class (salsa, flamenco, ballroom, disco, hip-hop, modern, jazz etc);
- Dancing to your favorite tune in your living room;
- Yoga;
- Pilates;
- Tai chi;
- Qi gong;
- Martial arts.

Investigate! Try something new out. Play with movement. Allow yourself to enjoy the experience of being in the body. It is not about pushing yourself to sweat and feel pain, it is about enjoyment and exploration.

Movement in the body can help the brain to produce feel-good hormones and chemicals, which reduce stress, anxiety and depression. Movement really can be mood altering and can improve our wellbeing, wellness and quality of life.

Taking time out each day to stretch your legs and move around in some way or another can be profoundly liberating. It is too easy to forget that this body is our vehicle on this earth and we often take it for granted. Getting out of our heads and out in nature can give us respite from continual thoughts.

✎ Take time to journal about your movement discoveries. Do you notice that movement has a positive impact on your mood? Do you feel excited about discovering new ways to move your body? Is there a new class that you feel compelled to try? Are you resistant to movement? Can you sit and hear what the critic or saboteur is saying? What is the resistance about? Is there fear of trying something new? Do you need support to help with this step?

There are other ways to explore being in the body too – such as osteopathy, acupuncture, massage, physiotherapy, chiropractic, reflexology, Rosen Method Bodywork, Shiatsu and many other complementary therapies! Anything that gets you feeling into your precious body is a great way to begin connecting your head to your heart and can help with reducing your emotional eating episodes.

Rambunctious resources for the exploration of movement

♥ Dr Christiane Northrup. *Women's Bodies, Women's Wisdom. The complete guide to women's health and wellbeing.*
♥ Local Yoga Class. Search UK: http://www.localyogaclasses.co.uk and

http://www.yoga.co.uk
- ♥ Pilates classes UK:
  http://www.pilatesnearyou.co.uk
- ♥ Tai Chi and Qi Gong classes UK:
  http://www.taichifinder.co.uk
- ♥ Dance classes in the UK:
  http://www.dancenearyou.co.uk and
  http://www.danceweb.co.uk
- ♥ To find a complementary therapist in the UK:
  http://www.embodyforyou.com

Chapter 17

The importance of being able to ask for support

It is easy to isolate ourselves from people and situations when we feel upset, stressed or tangled up in shame and guilt. As human beings we are naturally social creatures and, although time to ourselves can be cherished, it is also important to have people in our lives that we trust and who are there to support us and listen to us non-judgmentally.

Positive support on your journey of exploration into emotional eating patterns is a blessing and can also be a useful motivator. You need someone who you can speak to and say how you are feeling and what changes you are making. This individual needs to be someone who you can celebrate positive steps with!

Support comes in many forms: Good and trusted friends or family members, a therapist, counselor or life coach. An online support board can be useful too but sometimes it can lead to hiding behind a computer screen rather than actual, physical communication. You may be able to find a support buddy online who you can then speak to via Skype or the telephone. You might even find a complementary health practitioner who can be a support system for you.

🖉 How do you feel about asking for support? Who can you ask for support, or where can you go for support?

Being vulnerable and asking for support can be challenging, but love yourself enough to reach out, there are people who are waiting to support you on your journey!

Chapter 18

Spirituality and daily connection practice

When we don't take time to connect to our deepest wisdom it can often feel as though something is missing from our lives, it can feel as though there is a void and often we attempt to fill that void with food. Do you take time each day to connect with your deepest, most wise, real Self? This could be through journaling, sitting in silence for 15 minutes, meditation, prayer, a peaceful walk in nature, yoga, reading passages from nurturing texts, asking yourself the question, 'what do I really need?' or painting or drawing with no specific outcome other than to investigate your inner life.

🖉 How do you connect? Do you take time to connect? Could you make connection a regular part of your day?

Although things are changing, here in the Western world many individuals are unwilling to speak openly about 'spirituality.' There has been a move away from organized religion, which feels authentic for many people, myself included, but the yearning for depth and connection to 'something' is often still felt. Building a strong spiritual, or connection, practice can be incredibly healing. My upbringing involved a strong religious element. From a very young age I questioned this faith from every angle. For many years now I would not describe myself as religious in any way. Instead I have a deep-seated spirituality that I would not be without and I do believe that my upbringing helped plant the right seeds. The core of all religions is the same. LOVE. The message from my upbringing that I choose to hold on to, is 'love one another,' and 'to love thy neighbor as thy self,' and to experience the Divine within myself and myself as a piece of the Divine.

The meaning of spirituality

Spirituality is a really difficult word to define, and perhaps that's because it is above definition in words? Many people interchange the words 'religion' and 'spirituality' but there is a really huge difference between the two. Spirituality is not religion, although religion can include a deep spirituality. Personally I have a profound and deep spirituality but I am not religious at all.

Religion is an organized system of beliefs, practices, rituals and symbols, which can help a person to become closer to God/higher power etc.

Spirituality is more about the personal quest for understanding answers to questions about life, about meaning, about our relationship to the sacred or transcendent. Spirituality can certainly be closely linked to religion but religion is not necessary for spirituality.

Spirituality is about deepening awareness. The Sanskrit word Buddha originally meant 'awakening or 'coming to.' In his book *The Book Of Secrets*, Deepak Chopra writes about some of the questions that are often key to deepening our sense of Self, of spirituality:

> The most that any teacher can do is open the door; he can answer three questions in the age-old way:
>
> Who am I? You are the totality of the universe acting through a human nervous system.
>
> Where did I come from? You came from a source that was never born and will never die.
>
> Why am I here? To create the world in every moment.

The great philosopher Pierre Teilhard de Chardin, in his book *The Phenomenon of Man*, wrote, 'we are not human beings having a spiritual experience; we are spiritual beings having a human experience.'

Spirituality can be thought of as being an inner path enabling a person to discover the essence of their being.

🖋 What does spirituality mean to you? Do you have a spiritual connection practice, how does it impact your life? When you don't connect how does that impact your day?

Having a connection practice is a way to help us to develop our inner life, our spirituality, our interconnectedness with the whole; the whole of life, the cosmos, the ALL. It helps us to remember that we are not alone; we do not have to deal with struggle on our own. A connection practice helps us to develop compassion, forgiveness, love, harmony and other such qualities, which deepen our connection to life, beyond the materialistic.

Roberto Assagioli, the Italian psychoanalyst and father of Psychosynthesis psychotherapy devised the following dis-identification exercise as a way to help us to feel into our deeper, true nature.

Sit in a comfortable position; spend a few moments with your breath. When you feel relaxed read through the following paragraphs.

I have a body but I am not my body. My body may find itself in different conditions of health or sickness, it may be rested or tired, but that has nothing to do with my self, my real 'I'. I value my body as my precious instrument of experience and of action in the outer world, but it is only an instrument. I treat it well, I seek to keep it in good health, but it is not my self. I have a body, but I am not my body.

Close your eyes and reflect on what you have just read. When you feel ready open your eyes and continue:

I have emotions, but I am not my emotions. My emotions are

diversified, changing, and sometimes contradictory. They may swing from love to anger, from joy to sorrow, and yet my essence – my true nature – does not change. 'I' remain. Though a wave of emotion may temporarily submerge me, I know that it will pass in time; therefore I am not this emotion. Since I can observe and understand my emotions, and then gradually learn to direct, utilize and integrate them harmoniously, it is clear that they are not my self. I have emotions, but I am not my emotions.

Close your eyes and reflect:

I have a mind, but I am not my mind. My mind is a valuable tool of discovery and expression, but it is not the essence of my being. Its contents are constantly changing as it embraces new ideas, knowledge, and experience. Often it refuses to obey me! Therefore, it cannot be me, my self. It is an organ of knowledge of both the outer and the inner worlds, but it is not my self. I have a mind, but I am not my mind.

Reflect.

Now comes the stage of identification:

After dis-identifying myself from the contents of consciousness, such as sensations, emotions, thoughts, I recognize and affirm that I am a centre of pure self-consciousness, a centre of will. As such, I am capable of observing, directing, and harmonizing all my psychological process and my physical body.

Focus your attention on the fundamental realization: I am a centre of pure self-consciousness. Rest in this awareness. Repeat to yourself:

I recognize and affirm myself as a centre of pure self-awareness and of creative, dynamic energy. Beyond this 'I' is the ever present, pure consciousness, the Self that is one with all, of which 'I' am a reflection.

✎ What comes up for you when you do this exercise?

Learning to connect to our deeper, True Nature, is so powerful. From this place we can be more observant of our thoughts and feelings and we feel supported and more able to cope. Turning to food is a coping mechanism, which is dis-empowering. You are giving your energy and power away to an outside force, thinking that food can solve your problems and take away the pain. It is far more empowering to connect to your deeper Self, to not give your power away, to know that you are supported in this connection with your Self.

How do you know you are connected and it's not just another voice? When you are connected to your True Nature there is no criticism, no shoulds and cannots, you feel safe, empowered and supported. There is peace, there is calm, there is clarity. The choices you make from this space serve you in a loving and tender way.

Eating as a mis-interpreted call to live more in the body

When I was gorging myself on food I had a moment of realization. It felt as though my spirit was trying to get me to live a more embodied life. I was being called to feel my body more, allow myself to operate on this earth through the vehicle I had been given – my body. Food made me feel heavy; it really made me feel my physical body, something that I didn't usually feel. I had always felt as though I was living outside of my body, floating above it, or to the side. I wasn't so happy with being human. Through exploring my emotional eating I felt as though I was being called to live a different kind of spirituality, an embodied spirituality. I needed to learn to be rooted in the earth as well as swaying in the heavens. I had to ground my high ideals of spirituality into my body and my life on this earth.

It was something that I always struggled with, being human. I was always trying to escape, even as a child. Asking big questions that no one around me seemed to be able to answer and feeling intensely uncomfortable in this human skin was something that challenged me a great deal. I didn't recognize my own reflection and looking at photographs of myself always shocked and un-nerved me. My 'essence' just felt too large to fit into this skin. As a child I lived outside of my body, often viewing it from a distance, it is hard, even now, to describe. In my late teens and early 20s I began to meditate and became obsessed by transcending (even annihilating) the self. I wanted to be 'pure consciousness,' I wanted to stay in the state of bliss that I experienced in my meditations.

It pains me now to say that I hated having a body; I didn't want to be spirit operating through a human nervous system. I didn't want anything to do with being human in some regard, but on the other hand I had this huge, huge love that I wanted to give out to humanity. Confused doesn't even begin to describe it.

In my teens I experienced bouts of anorexia, not feeding this body and then, years later, ended up compulsively overeating and feeling my body on a deeply painful level. Something was always drawing me back to my body, calling me back. I studied for a masters degree in nutritional medicine – ironically that was all about the body! For myself personally, becoming ill (with lupus spectrum disorder) with an autoimmune disease was also a big wake up call. I had spent so long not wanting to be human that my body seemed to be mirroring, reflecting, my wishes and was shutting down. It was the call to begin the journey to loving this human self whilst retaining my connection to the Divine. I felt, like Caroline Myss quips, like 'a mystic without a monastery.' Yes, I still wanted to transcend the body, but in order to authentically grow, spiritually, I knew I had to include it too (not just shun it).

Whilst studying psychosynthesis (a form of counseling/ therapy) I realized that this human experience was actually a blessing because without this human self-consciousness I would simply 'be' pure consciousness and hence I wouldn't know the beauty of being able to actually experience it. An Indian sage once said, 'I want to taste the sugar, I don't want to be the sugar.' I'd go a step further and say that my desire is for both – I deeply want to be the sugar (pure consciousness) but I also want to taste the sugar (through my human self-consciousness). We are the emptiness and the manifestation, oneness, non-dual.

Now I seem to have settled into the knowing that I am self becoming more and more aware of Self, the true and essential nature of all, no separation, no duality. Finally I am coming to terms with, and embracing, my humanness. I love that I arise from 'what is' and that I have self-consciousness to be able to experience that. Suddenly I realize that life is heaven and I keep awakening and unfolding into that. When I let go of dualism there is no bad/good or right/wrong, there is what is without the struggle.

The growth will never end, it is a process. I feel like a star, as You are a star. I am a face like Your face. I am a reflection. The Source, the light, I am that too – but without this face, this image, this human mind I would not know my Self. This image, this projection, this emanation, it allows me to experience what is, it allows me to experience myself, Pure Consciousness, True Nature (or however you wish to refer to THAT).

Jack Kornfield expresses this eloquently when he writes in his book *A path with heart*:

In the depths of their silent listening many meditation students have discovered that from an early age their life experience was so painful they did not want to be born and they did not want to be here in a human body. They look to spirituality to provide an escape but where will the notions of purity, of going beyond or transcending our bodies, our worldly desires, our impurities lead us? Does it actually lead to freedom or is it only a strengthening of aversion, fear and limitation? Where is liberation to be found? The Buddha taught that both human suffering and human enlightenment are found in our own fathom-long body with its senses and mind. If not here and now, where else will we find it.

Spirituality isn't about losing yourself in religious dogma or rules prescribed by any self-help book, or teacher, or a course. Spirituality is about looking inside of your Self, to that wise place within. Of course, certain books and teachings can help us to connect to that place, but the wisdom is there for everyone, you do not have to follow one specific path. Look inside of yourself, look within the depth of your being and ask, 'Who am I?' Who is this ever observant I? It is about relaxing into the now of your own situation.

In terms of emotional eating, we need to relax into our body as our vehicle on this earth, yet remember that the body isn't all of who we are. Who you are, who I am, is so precious and at the core there is blissful, all-pervading awareness. Spirituality is about passion, creativity and joy and it is also about accepting the sorrows. It is about finding your peace in a situation, your own "I" of the storm, whilst the winds rage around you.

Sometimes accepting this body seems very challenging – but is it? Or is it just us bowing to outside pressure not to accept it? Often I find my body a challenge. There is often pain in my day from the lupus condition my body is currently dealing with. I have come to see that pain is not my pain, it is simply pain. There is pain all over the world. As I write this section I am also being challenged by the fact that I have painful cysts on my face. They look like acne. The voice of my inner critic kicks in – telling me I am too ugly to go out, that I should stay in and hide, that I need to wear a baseball cap, that I am not good enough, that I must be a 'bad' person, or dirty or whatever. I catch myself buying some more natural face-cream to use on my skin, hoping for a miracle cure. The real miracle would be to change my mind, to love myself anyway. To love myself more! I decide to sit still in silence, to connect. In that place I remember to anchor myself to the Divinity that I am. Nothing is wrong with me. There is nothing to say my skin is bad. Holding peace is healing. Yes, it hurts. Yes, I intend for these cysts to leave, but no, I am not bad or wrong. I have to hold onto my centre. It's ok. It is always ok.

We have to learn to relax with our bodies. If anyone outside of us is judging us it really doesn't matter. The question to ask is if you are judging yourself – because that is the real pain. So, in this moment accept where you are. Right now. At this particular shape and size. STOP. This is it for this moment. This is your starting place. You are changing and loving yourself more and you are starting now from where you are. How you are is not wrong. It simply is. As you love yourself more you will inves-tigate your feelings more, your need to squash your emotions and needs with food will lessen, and you'll start to eat in a way that is good for you. Your body may, or may not, change shape. Love yourself every step of the way.

Goddess bodies

Many years ago, all over the world from Greece to the Far East Women were revered and Goddess worship was normal. Women were honored because they give birth to new life, they signified the miraculous and the fertile. Goddess images also celebrate the diversity of women's shapes. There were Goddesses that were very large, with large bellies and breasts. Goddesses with small breasts and large thighs, tall thin Goddesses, all shapes and all sizes were celebrated. The female form, in all shapes and sizes, was considered sacred, Divine, holy. This is how we must treat ourselves now, respect our beauty and Divinity. Spirituality is not masculine or feminine, it is within all. It is the awareness that holds life, just as it is.

Poetry is one way that I connect, it represents a relationship with a deep part of myself. Most of my poetry was written during a time of deep searching. Each poem led me back to the Mystery of my Self, of that which is greater than me and yet embodied by me. A paradox beyond words. During this phase of seeking I found a deep solace, a feeling that I truly could be a great friend to myself at a time when old friendships were falling away and un-authentic romances seemed pointless. I recognized that when I was alone with my Self, I was never truly alone; I was the Mystery and the manifestations. The poems are my connection to Spirit; I reached down into my depths when they were written. I read them back at times and cannot remember writing them. They came through me as great waves, which I released, into words. None of my poems have titles, they are just free-flowing words:

Separate
Today I am separate
You seem too far away to touch
To feel
To taste
You left me cold
Outside
No way in
I scratch at the door
But it does not open
This pain of separation
Almost too hard to bear
But the glimmer
The glimmer of You in my heart
Keeps me from complete loss

* * *

It is all here
In my hands
My heart
It is all here
I bend down
I touch the earth – my skin
The ocean – my breath
The sun – my hair
I wear this cosmos as a cloak
I eat the stars
Off the tree of everlasting life
I sit with Jupiter in my knee
And Neptune on my shoulder
It is all inside my empty heart
Full with recognition
I taste You
And I see
This taste
Is me

* * *

I found You once
And You devoured me
I lay like minced-meat
In a pile
Ecstatic

* * *

My sensitivity feeds You
My hips

My belly
The broadness of my feminine thighs
My round cheeks
And my pert, small breasts
You take me all in
And honor the Mystery
No conformity here
No censor
Wild and juicy
I roam free
I am the sacred
The revered
The all
The only
Me

* * *

I ache for You
And when I am still I return
Back into Your embrace
To merge
As one that was never separated
The knower
And the known
The reflection
And the Source
Consciousness making love to consciousness
You cannot leave me
For You are it
And I am You
And in that knowing
Eternal peace

* * *

It is the way it always was
But with more acceptance
More light to cast out the shadows
It is the way it always was
But these eyes are new
My vision has changed
Everything is transformed
It's bizarre this feeling
This dualistic world
When I am wrapped in You
There is no separation
No label
No doubt

* * *

Merge with me
Two souls
Mingle
Become One
Destroyed
Become nothing
Everything
Vast
Miniscule
We are what was
What is
Before words were
Or are
I crave this annihilation

* * *

You speak to me so clearly
Yet my fears cloud your poetic embrace
I beg You for the answers
Then I turn to hide from pain
Lift me up and take me
Call my name
The burning
The yearning
My struggle torments my brain.
Keep me quiet
Still my racing mind
Plunge Your golden dagger
I'm your sacrifice
You're mine

* * *

I found You sitting there
Where You have always been
Accepting me as You have always done
You loved me even in my shame
You hold me even when my actions are insane
You light me up when I fall into my shadow
You see my clarity when all I see is my confusion
When I look at You I laugh at the absurdity I create
You never leave
You never try to escape
You are the core and the reality
You are the world
You are me
You could never abandon what is
You are the connection
The unconditional
The love that was and always will be

* * *

When You hold me in Your arms
And look into my eyes
Can You begin to conceive
Of the demise
Of separation?
When You inhale my laughter
Do You smile at the joke of a boundary?
When You enter the void
Of my limitlessness
Do You finally understand?
Can You lose yourself
In me?
Do You see
There lies the nothingness
That was
And always will be?
It was never a case
Of You
And I.
Can You expand
And go beyond
The concept of Infinity?
Can You dance up on the stars with me
And trust the possibility

Spiritual connection as a form of intimacy

Eating is an incredibly intimate experience. When we eat we are imbibing a substance, allowing it into our precious, physical body. This food is then taken into us and merges with our very cells, becomes part of our physical selves. It is difficult to think of anything more intimate than that. We allow ourselves to be physically transformed by the food we eat. Learning to get that kind of intimacy in a safe way outside of food is the challenge. Having a spiritual connection practice can provide that level of intimacy, a hug for the soul. Connecting to someone through a hug or meaningful conversation leads to all kinds of chemical reactions in the body and brain. Hormones are released, we feel good. Having a spiritual practice can produce that feel-good hit in a safe way and can open doors into untouched places of passion and knowledge, if we allow it.

In 2012, scientists proved the existence of something called the 'Higgs-boson' nicknamed the 'God Particle,' apparently a key missing piece for understanding how the universe words. This tiny, tiny, sub-atomic particle apparently forms a kind of energy field, the Higgs field, and as far as I can understand it, this invisible energy field pervades the universe like a cosmic treacle, as other particles pass through it they pick up mass, they get bigger, they gain size and shape and this allows particles to then form atoms which is what we, and everything around us, are made of. Apparently without these Higgs-boson particles, and the field they form, particles would just fly around space like light does.

So what? We didn't come to read this book for a quantum physics lesson, you might be thinking! No, you didn't, but think about it. We are all made of the same stuff. We are all inextricably linked. Strip us down to atoms and then sub-atomic particles and then teeny-tiny Higgs-thingies and we're all the same. We are all made of the same stuff. One Higgs-boson is not prettier than another, it's not fatter or thinner or this or that.

This isn't really my point anyway. To be fair, this discovery was pretty wild in physics terms, but 'God Particle,' really? For me the really BIG thing in all of this is the fact that what has been discovered is still a particle. Think about it, it's a particle, which means around the particle there is space. What's in that space? That's the true mystery isn't it? A particle still means there is separation. Still an outside and an inside. Still a barrier. The whole has no barriers and no space, it is all-inclusive, it is the awareness within which everything, including all the particles arise. It is the Emptiness that births the manifestations. We are all whole parts of a greater whole.

For me the beauty of this consciousness is what all the great wisdom traditions have always taught. We are all One. Zero separation. No space. A full-Emptiness. Being separate is an illusion but at the same time it's not because it is felt. The words of these traditions, the words of the Masters can seem strange and they don't seem to make sense, but that's because as soon as words are used to describe this awesomeness the mind gets involved and then comes confusion. What these great people attempt to describe in words is ineffable, it cannot be described in words, it is beyond words, beyond the intellect, beyond the mind. It is a felt experience of knowing.

What these teachings attempt to describe is the fact that there is no-where that Spirit is not. There is nowhere that isn't already fully enlightened. Enlightenment cannot be got, grasped, learned or gained because we are already THAT. Of course, we can evolve and grow and learn stuff but at each 'level of consciousness' we are, already, pure perfection, fully enlightened, realized individuals. No grasping is needed, in fact the more we grasp, the more elusive it all becomes.

Ken Wilber, my all time favorite philosopher/pundit, writes:

And so it is that we all inevitably end up feeling that we just can't see IT, no matter how hard we try. But the fact that we always can't see IT is perfect proof that we always know IT. That is, the very state of not-knowing Brahman is the Ultimate State of Consciousness, and that is exactly how you feel right now.

We are already that, we cannot see we are that, but deep down we do know it and we can certainly relax into it and feel it and be it.

Just rest, rest as the seer who cannot see itself, BE that. You know what? That, THAT state is more exciting than any particle, ever. Thinking too much about this can cause confusion and a messed up head! That is because as soon as the intellect gets involved it's all over.

Go back to the section on thoughts where we look at being the observer, the witness. Just BE that. BE IT as a felt experience rather than a thought about thought.

Writing so deeply about spirituality is like sharing an innermost preciousness, it's the kind of spiritual questioning that I grappled with as a child and had no idea how to put into words. Again you might be wondering 'what has that got to do with me?' You tell me, what has it NOT got to do with you? Even if you want to stick to the science, even then you have to admit, when all is said and done, we are the same, You and I, same particles, same Higgs-bosons holding us all together. So drop any body shape envy and comparison – because your Higgs-boson is not better than mine!

If you want to take it a step further. That observer, that witness who can observe everything except itself – that is YOU and that is ME. No difference at the core, no better, no worse, just 'what is.'

Instead of feeling into this knowing we seem to prefer to compartmentalize, we prefer to struggle. We prefer to label that as better than that. We prefer to call her bad and her good, just because she is thin and she is curvy, or vice-versa. Read again the words of Shylock from the Shakespeare play *The Merchant of Venice*, replacing the word 'Jew' with 'Woman'.

Hath not a WOMAN eyes? Hath not a WOMAN hands, organs, dimensions, senses, affections, passions? Fed with the same food, hurt with the same weapons, subject to the same diseases, healed by the same means, warmed and cooled by the same winter and summer? If you prick us, do we not bleed? If you tickle us, do we not laugh? If you poison us, do we not die?

Yes, you see, perhaps you're feeling me now. If we dropped the labels we'd have more love in our hearts, more compassion, and more equilibrium. Perhaps we'd stop beating ourselves up. We attach so much meaning and struggle to everything because 'just letting go' feels like a death, and a way it is a death, it's a death of the separate self and a falling into the arms of Oneness. Is sorrow really bad and happiness good? Or is sorrow just sorrow and happiness just happiness, without the attachment of a label, without the bad vs. good? Without the dualism. And is thin good and fat bad? Is overeating bad and controlled eating good? Or have we just lost the plot a bit?

Over the years I have read more than a few books, which suggest that if only we were more spiritual we could be saved from emotional eating. I say that is ridiculous. Being Spiritual does not mean we are let off the hook from being human! I have a deep, unwavering love of the Divine and I believe that there is nowhere that the Divine (God, Tao, Bliss, Love, whatever you want to call it) is not. Even in the midst of a full blow compulsive eating episode I know that the Divine is there, even that is enlightenment. Just letting go of the struggle of thinking that is bad brings sweetness back, it also brings awareness and means that perhaps next time there won't be a binge because you'll choose a move loving option for yourself.

The great Sri Ramana Maharshi, perhaps the greatest guru who ever lived, said something isn't a 'sin unless you believe it to be so' – I take this to mean, when the mind gets involved, when there is a question of duality – separation and labeling of bad and good – then there is pain. I believe that what we are is pure love. That never changes. That does not mean that we can indiscriminately go around doing hateful things – but when we remember we are pure love, Divine pieces, then we live congruently and the good/bad divide doesn't manifest because we become the mother of the split, we become the ground beneath it, we become what gives birth to the thought of good/bad and we can make a choice. When we forget who we are, when we forget we are love, when we forget we are Divine, it is then that we split and do things we later think were 'bad.' Loving ourselves is a step, an important one, to realizing we are pure love.

There seem to be a wave of New Age spiritual teachers who have an opinion about food and weight. A few of these women are incredibly thin and I wonder if they truly believe this is what we all need to be? Women are so different in shape, height, size, curvaceousness. Some of these teachers have written books about weight and there is wisdom there within those books, but the fact that they even mention weight makes me shudder. Weight is meaningless in the quest of a healthy, vibrant body. Yes, very slim women who weigh little are not going to be so healthy and women who are very large will also have health risks – but the point is, when we love ourselves, listen to the body about food, we will come to a place where we are a shape that doesn't change much, our own natural shape, a peaceful place. A natural balance. Weight loss is not the goal, weight loss it the by-product of self-love. The goal is to find deep love and respect for ourselves, as ourselves as spiritual beings, which means a respect for the whole of humanity. The by-product is that weight might be lost and shape may change. That doesn't mean everyone will be thin, it means that when we love ourselves, over time the body will find its natural balance. That natural shape will be beautifully unique and because we'll be choosing to vibrantly eat healthful foods and move our precious bodies it will be a healthy body too.

We are, each of us, a personal embodiment of the Divine. A certain weight or shape is not the goal. Inner peace is the goal; freedom from the obsession with food is the goal. Vibrant health is the goal – and this comes from trusting the inner Divine wisdom.

Many women, especially those who have begun to delve deeply into their interior and spiritual life, find that there is sometimes an essential feeling of 'aloneness' that can trigger eating. This seems to be a significant point to explore. It could be that we are tapping into a really important sense of knowing that we are 'all one' and actually more than that, we are all what was before one even came into existence, in this place there is a tinge of aloneness, of Emptiness. Emptiness with a capital E is used here instead of emptiness because there is a difference, Emptiness is full with life, everything emanates from that place of aliveness, and all manifestation comes from THAT. However, I think we often confuse that Spiritual sense of Emptiness with emptiness of the separate self, or ego, and so we reach for food to fill the void. Fearlessly feeling into Emptiness helps us to access a gateway to Spirit and we can learn to be, and in fact peacefully rest, with that which gives birth to this manifest world.

This is really difficult to put into words and for a fabulous account I would recommend reading an interview Ken Wilber did with *Pathways: A Magazine of Psychological and Spiritual Transformation*, which you can access freely via this link: http://wilber.shambhala.com/html/misc/pathwa_titoat.cfm.

In the interview Ken Wilber is asked why Spirit bothers to manifest at all, why does God incarnate? This is a great question, if we are all One, all emanations from this great Emptiness, why are we manifested in these separate bodies where there can be so much pain? Ken Wilber answers the interviewer with the answer given by many great Mystics, teachers and sages over the years, 'because it is no fun having dinner alone.' The One is manifested as the many, perhaps, perhaps because the One wants to experience itself through many faces? 'Ken Wilber: Doesn't that start to make sense? Here you are, the One and Only, the Alone and the Infinite. What are you going to do next? You bathe in your own glory for all eternity; you bask in your own delight for ages upon ages, and then what? Sooner or later, you might decide that it would be fun – just fun – to pretend that you were not you. I mean, what else are you going to do? What else can you do? Pathways: Manifest a world.'

As I became more connected to Spirit with meditation and other practices I began to rest as Witness, touching the feeling of One Taste, of being non-dual, a sense of no separation. With those experiences I also felt a sense of aloneness at times. The interview with Ken Wilber goes much further and deeper and makes a wonderful job of making some kind of sense of that which is ineffable. In 2006 I went travelling on my own. In Cuba, sitting on a mountain top I had a beautiful experience, difficult to word, I wasn't just looking out at the mountain scene, I was the scene, the clouds, the trees, there was no 'I' and as Ken infers above, there was also a twinge of feeling that there was no one to share it with.

Spirituality doesn't mean that suddenly our lives become perfect with no struggle

At the end of the day, the experience of One Taste, of Spirit, of Tao – is just that, a felt experience of freedom. Tapping into this, feeling Spirit, being One Taste, knowing your original face, the face you had before you were born, the face you had before the big bang – knowing THAT, feeling THAT, being that – doesn't automatically make life rosy! I used to think that if I touched Spirit, if I was a Spiritual being, then life would be easy and everything would be sorted out!! Ha, ha... it's like a Kosmic joke... In fact, I believe that being in touch with Spirit, holding One Taste and the knowledge of non-duality makes life deeper. I believe it makes us care more deeply, hurt more profoundly, cry more substantially, laugh louder, love harder and experience highs of ecstatic bliss. However, it doesn't mean that human problems vanish or that we don't still have jobs to deal with, financial strife, relationship issues etc. Matters of the world, of life need to be dealt with. Our own personal human neuroses do not vanish when we are spiritual, they still need to be investigated, unearthed, made more conscious, accepted as part of the whole. As we have seen with many spiritual individuals, priests, gurus, monks, nuns – they are still human and when human emotions are not dealt with these intensely spiritual beings are capable of human atrocities.

Having glimpsed Spirit and committed to a spiritual life we can either be motivated to be our best possible human self, to deal with our shadows and neuroses or we can get caught in an endless cycle of escapism, not wanting to deal with human issues. Being 'Spiritual' does not let us off the hook from life. As the brilliant M. Scott. Peck wrote as the opening line in his classic bestseller, *The road less travelled* – 'Life is difficult.' Being human is not necessarily easy, and being a conscious, Spiritual human, is still difficult, and perhaps more so because we are aware.

Don't get me wrong; I don't want to put a dampener on it! Being aware, being Witness, experiencing One Taste, living as non-dual, knowing THAT – adds technicolor to life and meaning and purpose and depth. It really is freedom. It can also be painful because we become aware of the destruction of humanity that could be changed if others were aware, awakened to Spirit, to Oneness.

The power of 'I AM'

Some call it 'the name of God' – 'I AM' is a powerful statement, an affirmation. Einstein said that thought was energy. It makes sense; everything that ever came into being was once a thought. It seems like a pretty good idea to think about dreams and what you really want to achieve rather than too much doom and gloom, although I totally think that it is a good idea to let stuff out sometimes, get it out of our heads and then move on to the positive. That's why I think gratitude is essential, as I have written about previously.

We all have our own sense of 'us' on this earth, and we can live that authentically, without the need to copy or conform. I rock a natural kind of spirituality. Hippy, free, me. However, for years (in my early 20s) I forced myself into a rigid spirituality because I thought it was what I 'should' do – there was a lot of fear around it, if I didn't do it 'right' I might get punished or I wouldn't achieve enlightenment! I was so strict with myself, I was evangelical about the fact that I didn't drink, I meditated for hours at a time, I exercised A LOT, I was incredibly strict with my diet and didn't wear jewelry or makeup and didn't think I was allowed to make myself attractive.

Spirituality was my beating-heart from a young age although I didn't know it was 'spirituality' then. I questioned everything that I was told about life, I had a painting of the black Madonna that winked at me; I had frequent out of body experiences and slept pushed up against the wall to make room for my guardian angel. The problem was I hated being human, I lived outside of myself.

After my relationship breakdown in 2006 I broke through. I began to allow myself self-expression. I drink the odd glass of champagne now and savor and love it. I walk and do yoga and cycle but not for calorie burning, pushing purposes but simply to feel and appreciate my body. Meditation is an integral part of my life – but I practice for 20 minutes to one hour a day instead of hours, I wear jewelry and sometimes makeup and I am in the ever-evolving process of loving my body. I trust mySelf. I continue to learn in this regard because sometimes I still feel like I want to escape. Sometimes I still find that being human is just not for me. However I take my daily steps and that for me is freedom.

There are no ideals when it comes to Spirituality. My good friend Lisa has piercings and tattoos and awesome lipstick and nails and her spirituality is incredibly important to her. Your own flavor comes from within. Find it. Hold it. Grow it. Evolve by following your truest wisdom.

I love philosophy and am in love with the words of Ken Wilber. I also have a passionate fascination with Sri Ramana Maharshi, he rocks my inner world. I practice meditation and I journal and do other things, but I don't have to do those things, spirituality is not about doing, it's about being. It is my deepest knowing that I Am already THAT, I have nothing to do to attain THAT.

Rigidity and spirituality don't mix. Rules are not necessary. It's about flow and fluidity. If you are used to dieting then you probably are used to rules, they make you feel safe, you think you are 'doing it right' although often you are ignoring your inner wisdom. Spirituality is about trust. Step off the diet hamster-wheel and into the arms of your Divine Self.

If you don't have a regular spiritual practice then I encourage you to try some out. Look for a local meditation or yoga class. Sit with your journal each morning and simply ask for wisdom and guidance. Open yourself up. Often when you ask, you are shown something.

People often ask me, 'Do you believe in God?' and I will always reply, 'depends on what your definition of God is.' A male ruler in the sky? NO. No I don't. An all pervading force, the mystery and the manifestations, the all and the nothing? YES. The primal song that resides at the heart of all hearts, YES. The ineffable that is both You and I? YES. If you want to call that God (or Goddess, or Tao, or Buddha Nature or Christ Consciousness, or Universe, or True Nature) then YES. What was before the big bang? YES. Not bound by time or space, I AM THAT I AM. YES!

An oak tree can be used to make a million different things. Each thing is its own, whole, individual, item e.g. a wooden spoon, but each item is also the Oak Tree. You and I and that stone and Freddy my dog and the earth and the shit and the flowers – all of these are individual, whole, manifestations, and all are God (of whatever you wish to call THAT).

Yes, spirituality can mess with the mind, precisely because it is beyond the individual mind. Drop the mind, go beyond and you'll see clearly, more clearly than you ever believed possible, and that is why spiritual practice is important, because it gets you off your head! Out of your mind, and in that place you will be able to see clearly.

If we all knew just how precious we were we would be on our knees honoring one another.

1. STOP. Breathe. Be here now. Feel.
2. Forgive yourself for whatever mistake you think you made. Start over.
3. Know that you are worthy.
4. Treat yourself as the Divine being that you are.
5. See that Divinity in others.
6. If you slip up go back to 1.

✐ Take time to write about any feelings, thoughts or sensations that came up for you whilst reading this chapter. Can you find a practice that feels safe to you now? Can you make time to connect daily? Does connection practice feel peaceful and helpful or does something else come up for you?

Rambunctious resources for the exploration of connection
(There are so many I cannot possibly name them all)

♥ http://www.dailygood.org/positive news
♥ http://www.beliefnet.com
♥ All books and resources by Caroline Myss.
http://www.myss.com
♥ Positive radio shows on Hay House Radio.
http://www.hayhouseradio.com
♥ You Can Heal Your Life online.
http://www.healyourlife.com

♥ Books by Jack Kornfield
http://www.jackkornfield.com
♥ Books by Cheri Huber
http://www.cherihuber.com
♥ Books by Thomas Moore
http://careofthesoul.net
♥ Books by Ken Wilber. He is deep; a good starting point is *Integral Life Practice* – his book written with Terry Patten, Adam Leonard and Marco Morelli. *Grace and Grit. Spirituality and healing in the life and death of Treya Killam Wilber* is also another beautiful book by Ken Wilber.

Congratulations!

Well done you gorgeous, courageous, beautiful woman. You took the step to explore your emotional eating patterns and have got to the end of the book. I am so incredibly proud of you. You crawled into your cocoon and began the self-exploration journey and I can see you now, beginning to emerge a changed person.

I'll tell you a little secret. You always were and are the most amazing butterfly. You just forget sometimes and step into the dream world of believing your thoughts and limiting beliefs. You can fly. You must fly and share your passions with the world. Butterflies come in all different colors, sizes and shapes and all need to be celebrated, and you can change your colors whenever you like, just explore and evolve and be positive and open to life. You are the witness to life and not the victim, that is an empowered position to be in.

In order to heal we have to choose to opt-out. Opt out from a society that doesn't include and celebrate different shapes and sizes. The only other option is to sell our souls to the diet-binge-obsession cycles. In that place there is no space to shine, to find and live your passion. It is a tiring place to be. To think about, and obsess about, our shape, size and food intake is exhausting. The goal here is peace and freedom from food obsession. The goal is to live more fully as you every day. From the very, authentic, core of you. Live it. That doesn't have to be extravagant, find your own flavor of REAL. Are you succulent, juicy, rambunctious, exuberant, sassy, sexy, hot, sensual, sensitive, nurturing, gentle, quiet, raucous or a combination of all things? Live that with no apology.

Do not be ashamed of your shadows. A beautiful painting would be nothing without shading and shadows; it is part of the whole picture. Our wholeness is just that, whole. We are not bad or good, we are real. When we deny a shadow and label it as bad it becomes powerful, it begins to get us to act out and then we punish ourselves with food.

Compassion for the journey

The poem below is a beautiful reminder to have compassion for your journey. We are human and we make the same mistakes over and over and over, until one day we awaken to what we are doing and we don't make the mistake any more. It takes courage to continue the journey in the face of constant stumbling, but it is worth continuing because the peace that comes with every step is SO worth it. When we are eating for comfort, and we know we are, it hurts us and at first we continue to do it even though we know it hurts us, this is the painful, painful part. However, we have to remember that we are always doing the best we can. Without the awareness of the habit we'd never be able to do it differently. As I re-read this poem I think of myself and the number of times I have fallen down the hole, but it has brought me to a place I would never, ever be otherwise.

Autobiography in Five Short Chapters
(There's a Hole in My Sidewalk)

Chapter 1
I walk down the street.
There is a deep hole in the sidewalk.
I fall in.
I am lost ... I am helpless.
It isn't my fault.
It takes forever to find a way out.

Chapter 2
I walk down the same street.
There is a deep hole in the sidewalk.
I pretend I don't see it.

I fall in again.
I can't believe I am in the same place.
But it isn't my fault.
It still takes a long time to get out.

Chapter 3
I walk down the same street.
There is a deep hole in the sidewalk.
I see it is there.
I still fall in ... it's a habit.
My eyes are open.
I know where I am.
It is my fault.
I get out immediately.

Chapter 4
I walk down the same street.
There is a deep hole in the sidewalk.
I walk around it.

Chapter 5
I walk down another street.

~ Portia Nelson

Delving into the black hole of emotional eating can plunge you head first into spiritual gold. Many women find themselves eating because they don't know what else to do. They say they are 'bored' – is this boredom a deeper dis-satisfaction with life? Sometimes eating can be used to block our dreams. We may have been taught that dreams were a waste of time, they couldn't become a reality. But all of reality was once a thought, a dream, an idea.

I'll say it again, who are you not to make your dreams real?

How often do you spend hours flicking through TV channels or do, do, do-ing and never taking time to sit in silence, to be, to hear the whisper of your own Self. Could you spend 15 minutes a day with your journal, just writing, or sitting in silence listening. Could you journal specifically about your dreams and what you'd love to do. Perhaps you are being called to go rock climbing, belly-dancing, to join a knitting circle, to walk in nature more, to cycle with your friend or partner. What does life whisper to you in the quiet moments?

Reading this book will not end your war with emotional eating, help you to lose weight or significantly change your life. No. Just reading this book won't do much. It isn't a magic wand, although I sometimes wish I had one. However, if you read this book, allow it into your soul, begin to trust your own inner wisdom, begin to love yourself – THEN, then I truly believe something deep within you will begin to shift. The power lies within you, not in the food you are eating and not within the pages of this book. You are so much more than what you think you are. It is time for you to begin embracing that.

If after reading this book you still find that you sometimes eat for comfort then do so with freedom and with love. Love yourself fully. No more beating yourself up about it. Use the book as a reminder. Go back and remind yourself to stop and breathe. Be mindful, remember that you can dis-identify from your thoughts, you can feel your feelings without fear. You are worthy of choosing to live the life that you desire. Your imperfections are all perfect. You are perfectly you – smiles, tears and all.

Start doing things for the love of doing them. Not because they make you money or may aid weight loss. Feed your soul.

Love yourself, celebrate yourself.

JUST LOVE

L.O.V.E. = LET OUTRAGEOUS VITALITY EMERGE

www.nurturewithlove.com

References

(1) Vaillant GE. 2011. The neuroendocrine system and stress, emotions, thoughts and feelings. Mens Sana Monogr. 9:113-128.

Tindle HA et al. 2009. Optimism, cynical hostility, and incident coronary heart disease and mortality in the women's health initiative. Circulation. 120:656-662.

(2) Tindle HA et al. 2009. Optimism, cynical hostility, and incident coronary heart disease and mortality in the women's health initiative. Circulation. 120:656-662.

**SASSY
BOOKS**

Hip, real and raw, SASSY books share authentic truths, spiritual insights and entrepreneurial witchcraft with women who want to kick ass in life and y'know...start revolutions.